YOUR
BEST
FACE
NOW

YOUR BEST FACE NOW

LOOK YOUNGER IN 20 DAYS WITH THE
DO-IT-YOURSELF ACUPRESSURE FACELIFT

SHELLIE GOLDSTEIN

AVERY
a member of
Penguin Group USA Inc.

Published by the Penguin Group
Penguin Group (USA) Inc., 375 Hudson Street, New York, New York 10014, USA •
Penguin Group (Canada), 90 Eglinton Avenue East, Suite 700, Toronto, Ontario M4P 2Y3, Canada
(a division of Pearson Penguin Canada Inc.) • Penguin Books Ltd, 80 Strand, London WC2R 0RL, England •
Penguin Ireland, 25 St Stephen's Green, Dublin 2, Ireland (a division of Penguin Books Ltd) •
Penguin Group (Australia), 250 Camberwell Road, Camberwell, Victoria 3124, Australia (a division
of Pearson Australia Group Pty Ltd) • Penguin Books India Pvt Ltd, 11 Community Centre,
Panchsheel Park, New Delhi–110 017, India • Penguin Group (NZ), 67 Apollo Drive, Rosedale,
North Shore 0632, New Zealand (a division of Pearson New Zealand Ltd) • Penguin Books
(South Africa) (Pty) Ltd, 24 Sturdee Avenue, Rosebank, Johannesburg 2196, South Africa

Penguin Books Ltd, Registered Offices: 80 Strand, London WC2R 0RL, England

ISBN 978-1-58333-440-9

Printed in the United States of America

Book design by Tanya Maiboroda

Neither the publisher nor the author is engaged in rendering professional advice or services to the individual reader. The ideas, procedures, and suggestions contained in this book are not intended as a substitute for consulting with your physician. All matters regarding your health require medical supervision. Neither the author nor the publisher shall be liable or responsible for any loss or damage allegedly arising from any information or suggestion in this book.

The recipes contained in this book are to be followed exactly as written. Neither the author nor the publisher is responsible for your specific health or allergy needs that may require medical supervision. Neither the author nor the publisher is responsible for any adverse reactions to the recipes contained in this book.

While the author has made every effort to provide accurate telephone numbers and Internet addresses at the time of publication, neither the publisher nor the author assumes any responsibility for errors, or for changes that occur after publication. Further, the publisher does not have any control over and does not assume any responsibility for author or third-party websites or their content.

ALWAYS LEARNING

PEARSON

Contents

Foreword by Rosanne Cash   vii

Introduction: One Amazing Journey   xi

1   Beyond the Fountain of Youth   1

2   Eastern Medicine and the Aging Process   14

3   Getting Your Best Face *Now*:
      The AcuFacial® Acupressure Facelift   34

4   What's Your Organ Type? Making Your Own Diagnosis   47

5   Puffy All Over: Welcome to Your Kidneys   54

6   Bags and Sags: Portrait of a Spleen Face   83

7   Dry and Withered Skin: Nourishing the Lungs   112

8   Hot and Bothered: Calming the Heart   144

9   Wrinkles and Sunspots: Love the Liver   170

10   Feeding Your Face the *Right* Way   198

11   Skin Care Rituals for a Fit Face   208

12   The Perfect Match:
      Finding the Right Practitioner for You   223

Appendix: Key Acupressure Points   229
Glossary   241
Acknowledgments   249
Index   251

Foreword

A FEW YEARS AGO, I WENT TO A DINNER PARTY at the house of some close friends, Gael and Stephen, whom I had not seen in several months. When I saw Gael, my jaw dropped. There was a remarkable change in her. She looked ten years younger than the last time I had seen her and her face glowed with a healthy, youthful radiance.

I examined her closely as we spoke. She definitely had not had a facelift. This was something deeper, something that came from a sense of wholeness in body and spirit, but on the surface her skin was as taut as a teenager's, and her color was luminous.

"Gael, what did you do?" I finally asked. "Did you go away to a spa for a few months or something? You look incredible!"

She smiled. "I've just been seeing Shellie regularly."

That night I vowed to see Shellie regularly myself, and it has changed my life. As a New Yorker, whose skin is exposed to noxious elements every single day, and as a woman with five children and a very full life,

I have tried every kind of bodywork, massage, scrub, facial, and decadent spa treatment ever invented. I love it all. They are all wonderful in their own way, and they can really take the edge off a hard week or soothe travel-ravaged skin.

But nothing compares to what Shellie Goldstein does. She works from the inside out. She has something very few medical practitioners or aestheticians have, which is equal parts knowledge and intuition, framed by a kind, nurturing presence and delivered with absolute professionalism, patience, and respect. She is a remarkable person, even without her great skill, but it is her knowledge of what creates true health and real beauty that is so special, and her ability to lead people to their own highest potential in both vitality and appearance that is so valuable.

Since beginning my work with Shellie (and it *is* work, a team effort of discovery and commitment), I have lost fifteen pounds off my body and ten years off my face. This is wonderful in itself, but the real payoff has been in the sense of well-being, the stabilization of hormone levels, and the energy increase I have experienced from the acupuncture, herbs, and her understanding of the most subtle energies of the body and how to capitalize on my individual strengths and mitigate my particular weaknesses.

This is the medicine and beauty ritual of the future, the treatment that goes beyond the surface and can remedy the sources, instead of the symptoms, of premature aging and disease.

Beauty is *not* skin deep. Beauty begins at the core of the person, and without genuine health it will deteriorate with age. Real beauty lasts a lifetime, and is the hallmark of vitality, strength, balance, and self-respect.

Every session I have with Shellie is exquisitely designed for exactly where I am on that particular day, and the work seeks first to find that balance, whether physical or emotional, then to heal and capitalize on my own health and beauty potential. Every woman has an inner beauty that can be suppressed and diminished by the hundreds of stresses of modern life, or can be gently discovered, supported, and released to rise to the surface of her visage. Shellie frees the captive beauty that we all hold hostage within us.

Catherine Deneuve once said that there comes a point in every woman's life when she has to choose between her face and her derriere, because the maintenance required to keep both in top shape is just too much.

I'm not sure this is true. Gravity and basic wear and tear are indeed immutable forces, but the energy field of a woman who knows herself and supports her intrinsic health and maximizes her beauty is a force of nature, and not entirely subject to gravity or time. I fully intend on keeping my face *and* my derriere in prime condition. But if forced to make a choice, I choose my face, and I'm turning it over to Shellie for safekeeping.

—Rosanne Cash

Introduction:
One Amazing Journey

LIKE SO MANY WOMEN OF MY GENERATION, I sailed through my teenage years with a love for fun and the sun. In my twenties and thirties, I ate what I wanted, stayed up late at night, and burned the candle at both ends—all while juggling work and my studies.

One morning after a late night of dancing and partying, I crawled out of bed after only three hours of sleep. I took a good, perhaps startling, look at myself in my bathroom mirror. Fine lines marked my forehead. My cheeks and jowls sagged. I was now in my early forties and showing it; the blemish-free glow of my thirties was gone. The flush of youth that I had always taken for granted was no longer visible to me. I suddenly felt like I was aging.

That was a turning point in my life—one of those lightbulb moments.

Recognizing that I was in desperate need of help, I sought refuge at the cosmetics counter—many counters, in fact—of my favorite department stores. Super and often expensive creams caught my attention with their seductive promises: Age Defying, Wrinkle Defense, and Age Reversing. They beckoned me from the shelves: "Boost your skin's anti-aging power," "Fine lines and age spots will disappear," "Sagging skin will miraculously tighten," "Deep wrinkles will dissolve," and poof, I will look ten years younger! I bought the claims—and the products. I quickly found out that most of them did *not* deliver what they promised.

So, armed with a master's degree in nutrition and a license in acupuncture as well as esthetics, I decided I could use my knowledge to address what was staring me in the face. While doing my research, I read that emperors and other members of the privileged class in China had been employing acupuncturists to enhance the youth and beauty of their concubines as far back as 960 A.D. It was the only anti-aging therapy I found that had such a rich history. It piqued my curiosity—and my interest. Modern acupuncturists like myself were not using their skills to address the cosmetic aspects of appearance.

Then opportunity knocked. I had the chance to go to China. While I was there, I observed Asian medical doctors treating patients suffering from facial paralysis with acupuncture and medicinal herbs. I saw highly trained specialists use acupuncture to relax and lift strained and flaccid face muscles and return them to normal. It was incredible to watch. Many of these patients commented afterward that they looked even better than they did before the paralysis had set in. I was intrigued by the success I was witnessing and ecstatic about the endless possibilities of using this knowledge to restore youth and beauty.

When I returned home, I delved deeper to find out more about how Chinese medicine sees and treats the aging process. In essence, Chinese medicine says we age from the inside out. What we see on the outside is a reflection of what is happening on the inside. Likewise, the visible signs of aging can be altered by treating from the inside out. If you are in better health on the inside, you're going to look better on the outside. I laid out a series of acupuncture points designed to address my own aging symptoms. My facial muscles lifted; my skin got smooth and was glowing again. I didn't look twenty, but I loved what I saw. My family and friends noticed the difference, too.

Then I started doing anti-aging acupuncture on my patients. I knew it would work, because it worked for me. Still, the results amazed me. The improvements I was making in the facial appearance of my patients were far beyond what I ever imagined. Not only did I witness age-reversing effects, my patients were experiencing improved health, less fatigue, more vitality, reduced stress, greater contentment, and increased focus.

Gradually I refined my technique to include Chinese herbs, dietary recommendations, and natural topical treatments. I got even more excited about the visible results I was achieving. I was decreasing fine lines and wrinkles, tightening sagging skin, strengthening weak facial muscles, improving skin tone, and reducing eye and facial puffiness—all by using acupuncture and food. No plastic surgery or Botox necessary!

My patients were ecstatic about their fresh and younger-looking appearance—their "secret" that had others wondering if they were getting some kind of invasive cosmetic treatment. It didn't take long before one patient told another patient, and that person told another. In no time, I could barely keep up with the demand for my unique age-reversing approach.

That was more than ten years ago. Today my practice is devoted almost exclusively to the rare subspecialty of cosmetic acupuncture, where I use my signature comprehensive AcuFacial® program to target age-related issues— especially as they pertain to facial appearance. In addition to acupuncture, I incorporate an advanced micro-current system designed by CACI International to improve facial muscle tone; ultrasound to remove unwanted surface skin, stimulate circulation, and drain sluggish lymph; and light-emitting diodes (LED), a kind of light technology that when applied to skin care can resolve acne, promote production of healthy collagen and elastin in skin cells, and improve overall appearance. A single session incorporating all of these state-of-the-art techniques can cost $500—hardly an expense that fits into the budget of most people. And that's where *you* come in.

After starting my AcuFacial® program, many of my patients were asking what they could do on their own to keep up their great new look, so I'd show them how to target the same points on the body that I had inserted with acupuncture needles by massaging them using acupressure. I started to notice that these people also seemed to be getting faster results than other patients. So I began showing all my patients how to perform acupressure and instructed them to do it between their weekly AcuFacial® sessions. My hunch turned out to be true. After several weeks, the patients who regularly used my acupressure technique were getting better and faster results than those who did not use it. I also noticed that the patients who performed acupressure on a regular basis between their monthly maintenance treatments not only were able to maintain the effects of their treatment longer, but also continued to show marked improvement. They had firmer muscle tone, tighter and smoother skin, and a softer, more luminous complexion.

Now it's your turn. The AcuFacial® Acupressure Facelift featured in this book is a natural self-administered facelift designed to mimic results similar to what people who come to me for my signature AcuFacial® treatment are achieving.

Your Best Face Now is the culmination of the past twenty-one years of my dedication to helping others look and feel their best. I don't promise to *stop* aging; no one can. I don't promise to take *decades* off your appearance, but, when properly performed, this program can erase years—*many* years—and will also help you feel your best. You *can* achieve your best face, and you can do it now, no matter what your age.

It is my hope that, unlike me, you don't have to find yourself staring at shelves crammed with false promises. *Your Best Face Now* is my promise that when you look in the mirror, you'll smile and love what you see.

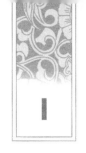

Beyond the
Fountain of Youth

of her facial wrinkles and the creases between her nose and mouth, and to firm her sagging cheeks. She had honey-colored shoulder-length hair and bright blue eyes, and was dressed in a classic black suit. She was in her early forties, but her face wore the lines of someone much older.

I noticed right away that her entire body was tense. Initially she stole quick, nervous glances at the acupuncture diagrams and posters on my office walls. She had never experienced acupuncture before, but had read in *Harper's Bazaar* about my trademark AcuFacial® technique and the value of acupuncture for enhancing facial appearance and improving overall health.

After Ann filled out a general health history form, we sat together to discuss her assessment of her facial condition and her desire for improvement.

"I'm only forty-three," sighed this classic multitasking married mother of two with a full-time job as the human resources director of a large firm. "I'm too young to have wrinkles, but I do. I looked at a photo taken four years ago at my parents' anniversary party, and I have aged so much since then. I think my harried lifestyle must be catching up with me."

I just smiled at the comment, as I had heard it from my patients so many times.

Ann's medical history revealed that she had no serious health risks, but she complained about mounting stress at work, difficulty sleeping at night, and other physical annoyances.

"I try to leave the office at the office," she said. "After I put the kids to bed, I usually have a glass of wine with my husband, we watch *Letterman,* and he's out like a light. I fall asleep fairly quickly, too, but then I wake up a few hours later. That's when my mind begins to race with every ridiculous detail I'm terrified I'll forget. From scheduling the kids' after-school activities, to deciding on a paint color for the living room walls, to whose turn it is to feed and walk the dog when I have to stay late at the office." She laughed. "I told you, ridiculous, right?"

"No," I said reassuringly, "your plate runneth over."

Ann reported that her overall energy level used to be good, but recently she experienced periodic bouts of fatigue. She noticed that after eating she often felt bloated and she complained about having gained weight over the past two years, despite regular workouts and frequent dieting.

"How much weight?" I asked.

"Eight pounds." She sneered. "I think my sister is secretly thrilled because I'd never had a weight problem."

"Let's get you on the acupuncture table," I said.

I made sure she was as comfortable as possible. The table had thick foam padding and soft covers. I placed a pillow under her knees for lower back support and one under her head for relaxation.

"I'm going to take a good look at your face to get an idea about what is going on with you—inside your body and out."

Using a powerful magnifying lamp that reveals what you can't see with the naked eye, the first thing I noticed was that Ann's coloring was pale with a yellowish cast. She had an oily T-zone—forehead, nose, and chin—with dry patches on her cheeks. Along the side of her left cheek were several light brown patches—sunspots from repetitive exposure to the ultraviolet rays of the sun. Though it appeared to Ann that I was trying to assess the extent of her cosmetic aging, what I was really trying to determine was her Organ type—not the organs recognized by Western medicine, but the Organs that are fundamental to Chinese medicine.

"Do you use sunscreen regularly?" I asked.

"I try," she said. "But I'm a sucker for a tan."

I also detected the first signs of muscle tone loss in her cheeks, jaw, and neck area. In addition to the deep crease between her eyebrows, I noticed several fine lines across her forehead.

"How much water do you drink a day?" I asked. Her eyes brightened. "I buy a huge bottle of water every morning and try to finish it by the end of the day," she said proudly.

"Good," I responded.

"Although," she continued, "sometimes, if it's crazy busy at work, I notice I've forgotten the water completely and find myself sitting through meetings drinking diet soda."

"What about coffee?" I asked.

"Only in the morning. One grande double cappuccino." I was beginning to get the picture and intuitively knew the answer to my next question without asking.

"Do you crave sugar?"

"All the time," she replied.

I clasped her wrist gently and explained that I needed to check her pulse. Similar to the radial pulse a Western physician takes to measure heart rate, an acupuncturist takes the pulse in six positions on both wrists to measure the health of the channels associated with the body's Organ systems.

"How's my heart?" she asked.

"Still beating," I joked, not wanting just yet to explain that I was checking more than just her heart rate. We both laughed, and I sensed that her anxiety was diminishing.

I found Ann's pulses were thin, full in the middle position, and deeper in the lower position. This revealed to me that she had a significant deficiency in the Chinese medicine field of energy known as Qi (pronounced *chee*), her Blood that flows with Qi was deficient, and her Organs were out of balance.

"Now, I need to take a look at your tongue," I said. According to Chinese medicine, the tongue is the visible end of a long tube that extends from the mouth to the rectum. Examining the quality of Ann's tongue—the size, color, texture, coating—would help me determine the condition of her Organs.

Ann's tongue revealed a lot. It was pale and puffy, had a wet white coating in the center, and the tip was slightly red with small spots. The paleness and swelling confirmed a Qi and Blood deficiency. The coating in the middle of her tongue was indicative of a digestive disorder. The spots and redness on the tip of her tongue indicated anxiety and related to her sleeplessness, and its overall appearance was a clear indication of the state of her Organs. Here is what I knew about Ann so far. She had:

- Fine lines and deep creases on her face
- Decreased facial muscle tone
- Pale, yellowish skin color
- Sunspots
- Difficulty staying asleep
- Bouts of fatigue
- Sugar cravings
- Bloating and other digestive issues
- Weight gain

A More Gentle, Natural Rejuvenation

Because Ann was new to acupuncture, I needed to explain my diagnosis in a manner that she could easily understand. The concepts and language of Eastern medicine, for the most part, are foreign to a Westerner's vocabulary and experience. In general, Western medicine does not differentiate between the cosmetic treatment of aging and the general health concerns related to the aging process.

Western medicine would view Ann's cosmetic problems simply as the result of aging, overexposure to the sun and other environmental factors and, possibly, a genetic predisposition to jowls, wrinkles, and a combination of dry and oily skin. A cosmetic surgeon probably would consider injecting botulinum (Botox), the drug made from the same bacteria that can cause dangerous and life-threatening botulism, into the deep crease between Ann's eyebrows, and adding fillers in the crease between her nose and mouth. He also might suggest a full or partial neck or facelift for her sagging cheeks and jawline. None of the other issues that Ann and I talked about would be of concern to a cosmetic physician.

Would Ann look better? Yes.

Would she feel better? Yes—about her facial appearance.

However, her sleeplessness, fatigue, weight gain issues, digestive problems, and food cravings would remain. To address these health issues, Ann would have to go to a doctor for a prescription for her sleeping problem, possibly another to get medication for her digestive difficulties, a third to address her lack of energy, and maybe even a fourth to lose weight.

A cosmetic acupuncturist would address them all. Why? Because they are all interrelated.

In Eastern medicine, the cosmetic signs of aging and physical health symptoms are not haphazard or coincidental. They are one and the same and can be traced to a deeper underlying condition—a weakness in one or more of five Chinese Organ pairs. Eastern medicine calls these weaknesses *patterns of disharmony,* and they represent the physical, emotional, and/or spiritual imbalances that prevent us from looking and feeling healthy and energetic. From the perspective of Chinese medicine, Ann's physical symptoms and the way her face was aging pointed to specific Organ imbalances caused by deficiencies of Qi and Blood.

"Ann," I began, "you have a weakness in a vital form of energy that we call Qi."

Her eyes widened. "Is that bad?"

"It's not bad, but it's not great. It's one of the reasons you're not looking and feeling your best."

I explained that Qi is a powerful force of energy, which you can neither see nor grasp, that travels throughout the body's Organ systems via invisible pathways called Meridians. To better help her understand the existence of Qi, I likened it to the flow of electricity through a network that allows light to fill a room.

"Think of the electrical current as Qi and the wires as Meridians," I said. "Your vital energy is not flowing optimally. Metaphorically speaking, your lights are dim. It's the reason your skin is pale and yellow, you feel bloated after you eat, and why you have trouble staying asleep at night."

"What about my wrinkles and sagging skin?" she asked.

"Those, too, are related to your Organ imbalance, Qi deficiency, and an insufficiency of Blood," I responded.

She looked worried. "Do you mean I need a transfusion?"

I smiled. "It can be a difficult concept to understand, but the answer is no. The Chinese concept of Blood is different from the blood you see when you cut yourself."

I explained that certain common medical terms used by Western doctors, such as blood and organs, are viewed differently in Eastern medicine. Blood is a form of energy similar to Qi that travels through the Organs and Meridians along with Qi. Although it, too, cannot be seen, it is important because it keeps our internal environment moist and our skin soft and supple. "When Blood is lacking, your skin looks dry, wrinkles develop, and you feel tired," I said.

In Eastern medicine, Organs are viewed as more than an anatomical mass. Rather, they reflect a complete set of specific functions that encompass the physical, emotional, and even spiritual. Qi and Blood course through these Organs along Meridians in a continuum, creating a Circle of Life.

There are specific sites on the body, called acupuncture points, that are aligned along the Meridians. By placing tiny, hair-thin needles into these points, it is possible to get Qi and Blood flowing properly to an Organ or Organs that are out of balance. This is how an acupuncturist treats disease and how a cosmetic acupuncturist helps erase the signs of aging. When deficiencies in specific Organs are addressed, the Circle of Life is renewed, and so is your internal health and external appearance.

Ann furrowed her brow, still a little confused.

"I know it's a lot to take in," I said. "The best way for you to understand is to let me give you a treatment and we'll see how you feel."

"Do the needles hurt?!" she blurted.

I patted the table gently and asked her to lie back down. "Some people feel nothing at all. Others, a tingling, or a slight prick. I'm told I have a light touch. Don't be surprised if you fall asleep. Many people find acupuncture extremely relaxing."

I quickly inserted three sterile stainless-steel needles into the surface of each leg. I then inserted two needles into each arm.

"Okay so far?" I asked.

"I barely feel them at all," she answered.

Next, I inserted five more needles—one in the center of her chin, one in each cheek, one on the top of her head, and one between her eyebrows.

"What does the one between my eyebrows do?" she asked.

"It helps you to relax."

She took in another deep breath. "Okay . . ."

"Think of this as nap time," I said.

I dimmed the lights, put on some soft music, and left the room. Ten minutes later I checked in on Ann. She was fast asleep. When I returned twenty minutes later, I gently roused her. Her eyes popped open. "I feel as if I just slept for eight hours."

I removed the needles and handed her a mirror. The tension in her face had disappeared, her skin tone was pink, and her bright eyes were clear and calm, as if she'd just returned from a trip to a health spa.

I worked with Ann, using acupuncture to balance her Organs, Qi, and Blood, and instructed her on a diet that complemented her Organ type and would minimize the possibility of future Organ weaknesses. I showed her an acupressure routine she could use at home and I adjusted her skin care regime to address her facial issues and condition. After ten weekly sessions, Ann's complexion looked healthy, even, and rosy, the fine lines on her forehead had disappeared, and the deep crease between her eyebrows had softened considerably. In addition, the muscles of her cheeks and jaw had tightened. Ann's energy was stable—no more bouts with fatigue—and she was able to easily sleep through the night. She no longer craved sugar, her digestion improved dramatically, and to her delight, she lost five pounds. Her coworkers and friends were convinced that she had undergone some kind of cosmetic surgery.

Your Best Face Now: The 20-Day Promise

Now it's your turn to get Your Best Face Now. And just as I did with Ann, I'm here to guide you all the way. The only difference is that you'll be doing acupressure, a Chinese medicine technique that you can do at home, instead of acupuncture. Acupressure works the same as acupuncture, but you use a finger or your thumb, rather than needles, to apply pressure to the specific points along the body's Meridians. Both acupuncture and acupressure are ancient Chinese healing techniques that have been acknowledged for their effectiveness by Western medicine and supported by thousands of scientific studies around the world. The National Institutes of Health database offers more than five hundred studies on the use of acupressure in the treatment of dozens of conditions, from hiccups and constipation to allergies, chronic fatigue, and insomnia, to musculoskeletal disorders, heart disease, and stroke. And a large-scale survey by the Centers for Disease Control and Prevention found the majority of Americans seeking health-related treatment over a one-year period chose some form of alternative medicine, including acupuncture and acupressure.

The results you will get using the techniques in this book will take a little longer to appear than they would with acupuncture, but if done properly and practiced daily, you should see changes in the way you look within twenty days. You should also notice an improvement in your health. All it takes is twenty minutes a day. Acupressure is easy to do and easy to learn.

The heart of this book is the twenty-minute-a-day AcuFacial® Acupressure Facelift, which is designed to rejuvenate your appearance by:

- Reducing wrinkles and deeper creases
- Eliminating fine lines
- Lightening dark circles under your eyes
- Decreasing eye and face puffiness
- Lifting sagging muscles in your cheeks, chin, neck, and brow
- Improving the quality of your skin
- Renewing a radiant and rosy glow to your skin
- Restoring the sparkle in your eyes

This natural facelift will erase *years* from your appearance. As with Ann and my other patients (as well as the women and men you'll read about in this book), people will look at you and wonder what you've "had done." What my clients say they like the most is the natural radiant look that shows they are aging gracefully and beautifully (or handsomely) in a way that defies their years.

People in their forties, fifties, sixties, and even older tell me time and again that they don't desire to look like a kid again; they just want to look (and feel) younger. They say they like the way they look and don't mind a few wrinkles, but are seeking something natural that will help them to restore their once youthful appearance. Many of my patients eschew invasive medical cosmetic procedures, even if they can afford them, because they worry about the pain and possible side effects. Although many people in general are happy with the results of cosmetic surgery, in recent years the trend has shifted to a desire for a more natural look. People are also hesitant about getting injections of botulinum, which not only is unnatural but can be poisonous if the dose is too strong. Besides, these treatments are only temporary and must be repeated at a steep cost every several months.

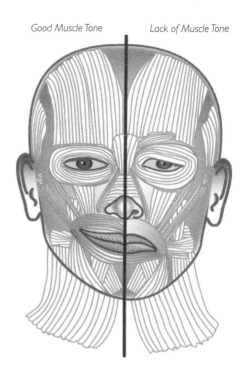

Good Muscle Tone   Lack of Muscle Tone

Acupressure is as old as Chinese medicine itself, dating back centuries. However, my AcuFacial® Acupressure Facelift is unique, as it is designed after my signature AcuFacial®, a natural facelift that incorporates acupuncture, micro-current to strengthen face muscles, ultrasound, and light-emitting diode (LED) therapy to repair damaged skin. Diet and a skin care regimen are recommended to help enhance the treatment. *Your Best Face Now* brings this technique from my treatment room to your home at a fraction of the cost. In fact, it can cost you virtually nothing, as I offer effective skin care formulas that you can make at home using common ingredients found in your kitchen. The handful of costly products I recommend I consider to be la crème de la crème.

The AcuFacial® Acupressure Facelift is effective because of the *way* it works.

Take a look at the diagram of facial muscles above. The left side illustrates the face of youth—strong muscle tone around the eyes and mouth, and in the cheeks. The muscles of the forehead and neck are elongated and relaxed. The right side shows the muscles of an aging face. As you can see, the muscles around the eyes and mouth are asymmetrical, the cheek muscles are droopy, and the forehead and neck muscles are too tight.

Both Chinese and Western medicine agree that wrinkles are formed from repeated muscle contraction. However, Chinese medicine takes it one step further and blames wrinkles on your faulty Organs. The two take a different approach to correcting the condition.

Plastic surgeons take the Western medicine approach by addressing the symptoms—wrinkles and sagging skin—rather than treating the problem—loss of muscle tone and your Organ imbalance. The plastic surgeon's approach is to separate the skin from the muscles, remove excess fat, pull the loose skin tautly over the muscles, trim the edges, then carefully stitch it back together. The result is tight, wrinkle-free skin, but the underlying muscle tone is still lacking. You end up with smooth skin over muscles that are either flaccid or too tight.

The Eastern medicine approach is quite different. A cosmetic acupuncturist targets specific acupressure points on Meridians to lift, tone, and balance muscle integrity, improve skin quality, and restore Organ health. The result is toned face muscles, reduced fine lines and deep wrinkles, refined skin and pore size, plus improved vitality and well-being. This approach also addresses many other concerns that you'll read about in this book.

The photos below illustrate the results that can be achieved through acupuncture and acupressure.

The photo on the left is the before picture of a forty-year-old patient with deep creases between the eyebrows and weak, sagging cheek muscles.

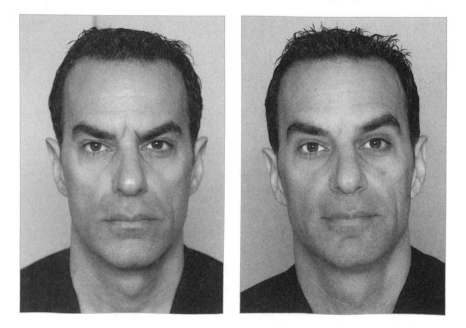

On the right, after ten acupuncture treatments, his wrinkles have markedly decreased and his muscles are toned and lifted. As a result, his appearance is softer and more open.

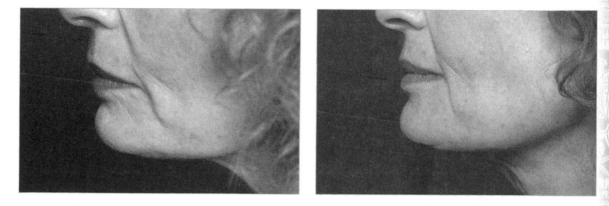

The photo above shows a sixty-year-old patient with sagging skin, a condition often attributed to loss of collagen and elastin in skin tissue. After ten acupuncture treatments, her skin is much plumper and appears more youthful.

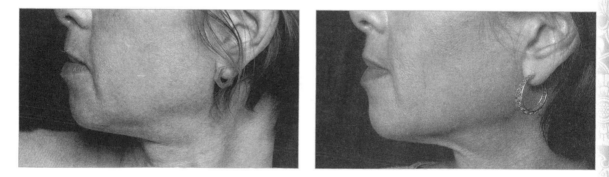

The photo above shows a fifty-one-year-old woman with a loss of definition along her jawline. After ten acupuncture treatments, her jawline appears much tighter and more defined.

How to Use This Book

Aging happens. We can't avoid it. But you *can* look terrific at *any* age. *Your Best Face Now* is designed to make it happen. It is my intention with this book to help you find your optimal approach to beauty and provide you with the necessary knowledge to enhance your facial appearance *and* improve your health.

Your Best Face Now is both curative and preventive. It is based on the principles of Chinese medicine as they apply to your appearance. Chapter 2 delves a bit into this philosophy to give you a basic understanding of Qi, Blood, Organs, and other elements discussed in this book and their impact on the way you look and feel. It is an important read for understanding why this program works. Chapter 3 is the heart of the book, the step-by-step illustrated AcuFacial® Acupressure Facelift. Follow the routine daily for twenty days and I guarantee that you—and others, too—will see a difference.

We all age differently because we have different imbalances in one or more of our Organs—that is, we're susceptible to certain weaknesses that cause some people to get pronounced droopy jowls, others to get deep creases in the brow, and yet others to have uneven and large pores, and so on. These strengths and weaknesses determine your Organ type. Knowing your Organ type means that you can optimize your beauty regimen with specific acupressure treatments, diet, and beauty recommendations. It's an added benefit! It generally takes a trained acupuncturist or Chinese medicine expert to pinpoint your Organ type. However, Chapter 4 offers a questionnaire that will help you figure out your personal Organ type.

Chapters 5 through 9 are profiles of each of the five Organ types—Kidneys, Spleen, Lungs, Heart, and Liver. These chapters offer insight into each Organ type's strengths and weaknesses and how it affects the way you look, age, and even act. The chapters also offer acupressure routines tailored to the facial needs of each Organ type that can be used on their own or in addition to the AcuFacial® Acupressure Facelift. In addition, you'll get important guidance on food choices, including recipes, that complement your Organ type and skin care choices.

What you eat plays an intricate part in the way you feel, and Chapter 10 reveals the ancient secrets of Eastern culinary wisdom. It also offers complete food lists that will help you eat according to your Organ type. And you don't have to roam the back alleys of Chinatown to find the ingredients. The foods that you will learn about can be found in most markets and grocery stores.

Chapter 11 offers a daily skin care ritual to optimize your AcuFacial®

Acupressure Facelift. It suggests time-tested, healthy product selections specifically for your skin type.

After you read this book, you may want to see an acupuncturist yourself. Chapter 12 leads you in the right direction.

The Appendix gives you a quick guide to the forty-six pressure points featured in this book and their specific benefits. If you have a special cosmetic problem or health issue you want to work on a little harder, you can apply acupressure to any of these points as often as you'd like.

It is said that the eyes are the windows of the soul. I believe that the face reflects the health of your body, inside and out. Follow the directions and suggestions in this book, and it will do wonders for the way you look, the way you feel, and for your confidence and self-esteem. With my decades of experience reflected in this book, you can have your best face now and every day, no matter what your age.

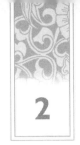

2

Eastern Medicine and the Aging Process

A WISE MENTOR OF MINE ONCE SAID, "YOU ARE not aging, you are growing." What a wonderful way to look at yourself! Instead of viewing the passage of time as a process of losing our youthfulness, we can look at it as a process of gaining—wisdom, confidence, contentment, and, hopefully, insight into what matters most.

There are many ways to view our aging selves, but for the purpose of understanding *Your Best Face Now* and why its program works so effectively, we need to look at aging through the eyes of Eastern medicine.

Beauty from the Inside Out

Think of all the times you have said or heard the expression "You don't look your age!" In Eastern medicine, a comment like this would be interpreted as meaning "You look to be in magnificent health!" This is because Eastern medicine sees your physical appearance, muscle tone, and the quality of your skin as a reflection of the health inside your body. Unlike Western medicine, Chinese medicine does not draw a line, even a fine one, between bodily health and cosmetic appearance. In Chinese medicine, health means more than our physical well-being. It encompasses everything about our persona—the state of our physical being, our emotions, our personality, how we think, how we act, and even our spirituality. It is why, as you noticed in Chapter 1, I asked Ann so many questions about herself.

Eastern and Western medicines view health, sickness, and beauty from different standards of beliefs. If you go to your dermatologist because you have acne, the doctor most likely will give you a topical skin wash or cream and a prescription for a medication to make the blemishes disappear. *Why* you have acne is rarely the focus of your visit.

If you go to a Chinese doctor because you have acne, you will be treated systemically for an Organ imbalance. You will be asked questions about your skin, and also about your diet, breathing, exposure to cold or hot air, your energy level, quality of your sleep, your moods, digestion, and bowel function. An Eastern practitioner will not only look at the skin on your face but also examine the skin on your body. He or she will look at your tongue and feel your pulse. You'll be asked to breathe in and out. You may also be asked questions about the health of your parents and siblings.

Eastern medicine sees wellness and illness through your Organ systems and the quality of Qi and Blood that run through them. In essence, it's all about *balance*. When your Organs are in balance, then so are your body, mind, and spirit—and it all shows in your physical appearance. Your face is the mirror of the quality of Qi and Blood surging through your Organs in and around a complex network of passageways known as Meridians.

EAST VERSUS WEST

There are many medical terms Eastern and Western medicine have in common, but they share little or no commonality by definition. To distinguish between the two, all references to Eastern medicine and its healing concepts are capitalized in this book. For example, heart refers to the organ beating in the body, but Heart is one of the twelve Chinese Organ systems.

When I think about Chinese medicine, it often brings to mind images of the movie *A River Runs Through It*, starring Brad Pitt, and the scene where Pitt's character is fly-fishing as his little brother quietly watches. There is a palpable, almost sacred energy in the movement of the water—the dancing of the light as the sun sparkles across the strong current and the fluidity of Pitt's character as he casts his line. The grace of his arm, the poetry in his hand, and the rolling stream of the river create a rich and endless flow, all one in harmony. This is the essence of nature and the fundamental principle of Eastern medicine: Balance (Yin and Yang), Movement (Qi), and Flow (Blood).

Yin and Yang: Maintaining Balance

Even if you aren't familiar with Chinese medicine, more than likely you are familiar with the terms Yin and Yang, which represent the meeting and harmonizing of two opposing forces. They are polar opposites as different as light and dark, hot and cold, summer and winter, wet and dry, birth and death. Yin and Yang represent powerful forces of motion, or energy. Like air and wind, you cannot see them, but you can feel their effects.

Yin symbolizes all that is dense, heavy, and earthbound. Like a tortoise, Yin is slow, methodical, and steady. It is cold in taste and feeling, quiet and tranquil in sound and manner. Yang expresses all that is light, porous, or ethereal. Like the hare, it is rapid, swift, and sometimes erratic. It is hot in taste and feeling, loud and energetic in sound and manner.

Yin and Yang energy blend as one in constant movement throughout your body and continuously adapt in order to maintain balance, like two children on a seesaw. Yin energy prevents Yang energy from moving too quickly and flying out of control, while Yang motivates the movement of Yin and prevents it from becoming sluggish or too bogged down. It's a delicate balance. Too little Yin or too much Yang moves you from a state of balance to one of imbalance. It manifests internally in many ways, ranging from one or more of many digestive woes, to minor health issues such as colds and headaches, to serious illness such as heart disease or cancer. Pain, for example, can be from an excess of Yang. Heaviness and swelling in your muscles can indicate too much Yin.

For followers of Chinese medicine, this is a well understood and accepted concept. What surprises many is the profound effect it has *externally* on the way your face changes as you age. When you are out of balance, the trained eye can see it in your skin and muscle tone. Wrinkles between your eyebrows and deep creases on the forehead may be a sign of too much Yang. Jowls, frown lines around the mouth, and sagging cheek muscles may be symbolic of not enough Yang. Spots on your face may signal too much Yin. A red, irritated complexion can represent not enough Yin.

Simply put, beauty and health occur when Yin and Yang are in balance. Visible changes occur when you fall out of equilibrium. Each of us is like a tiny universe made up of constantly shifting life forces trying to maintain the delicate balance.

The black and white sides of the illustration on the right represent the opposing forces of Yin and Yang. The dark half represents Yin and the light half is Yang. As you can see, there is a little Yang in the Yin half, and a little Yin in the Yang half. This is because they rely on each other for perfect harmony. Yin and Yang flow in a continuous circle, one moving into the other to create complete balance.

It All Revolves Around Qi

Balance, or harmony, is maintained by the steady flow of energy throughout the body known as Qi. This is the heart of Chinese medicine and the symbol of life itself. It is a powerful invisible force that cannot be seen, touched, measured, or isolated, yet it is ever present in all manifestations of life. Its movement shapes our physical identity, our thoughts, our moods, our actions, our spirituality, even the food we eat and the air we breathe. Every breath we take, every movement we make, encompasses Qi. It keeps us alive; without it, we die.

Like air, the quality of Qi is everything. When Qi is healthy, it moves freely like a summer breeze. When it is congested, it is oppressive and stagnates like smog hanging over a polluted city. When it is irritated, it whips like a tornado, creating chaos wherever it touches. When Qi is in good health, you feel your best and look your best. When your Qi is not moving properly, you can have aches, pains, and digestive upsets. You can feel sluggish, and you probably look and feel older than you should.

Qi is Yang. True to the nature of Yang, Qi motivates and moves you.

But it does not move alone. It stays in balance by moving through your body with another substance, known as Blood.

Blood: Qi's Counterpart

Blood, too, is visceral, though it is an easier concept to grasp because it is liquid and akin to the blood Western medicine sees running through your veins and arteries. Blood is Yin, and its primary purpose is to circulate and moisten your body and Organs. In keeping with the principles of Yin and Yang, Blood controls the energetic movement of Qi—not too fast to spin out of control, and not too slow to stagnate. Together they epitomize the harmony of Yin and Yang. Blood and Qi—Yin and Yang—flowing in tandem, keeping you in balance.

Moisture Is a Must

Moisture is intrinsically involved in Qi and Blood. It is composed of fluids in many forms—from the food and beverages we ingest and the tears, mucous, saliva, and sweat we secrete. Blood and moisture are on the same continuum—both liquid, both Yin—but they differ in the way they nourish the body.

Blood runs deeper in the body and its effect is stronger. Fluids circulate along the surface of the skin. Their job is to moisten—hair, skin, membranes, orifices, and flesh. Fluids also lubricate muscles, joints, the brain, and bones. Disharmonies of the fluids include dryness that we can see or feel on the lips, skin, eyes, and hair.

Jing: It's Your Essence

There is a fourth phenomenon in Eastern medicine called Jing, or Essence. Jing is your Yin and Yang essence. It is the embodiment of Qi and Blood; it cannot exist without them. Essence is *you* and distinguishes your individuality. It is the culmination of who you are and your potential for being. Essence comes from your genetic inheritance, the nutrients in the air you breathe, the foods and beverages you consume, and the lifestyle you lead.

As you age, your Essence dissipates. When it is gone, life ceases to exist.

Shen: The Window of Your Soul

Chinese medicine recognizes a fifth fundamental substance, called Shen. Shen is similar to your spirit. It is the force that determines your consciousness, your personality, your ability to think, discriminate, and act appropriately. Shen starts the movement of Essence and Qi.

Like Essence, you inherit Shen from your parents, and it is nurtured by the foods and beverages you consume, your lifestyle, and your attitude about life. Some say that the state of your Shen is reflected in your eyes. Sparkling eyes are indicative of a healthy Shen. When your eyes are dull, lack luster, or appear angry, it possibly means that your Shen is disturbed.

Chinese Organs: Stations of Operation

Qi, Blood, and Essence are produced and stored in our Organs as visceral bundles of energy that circulate through and around the body. They are like the body's operating systems that function in tandem to keep you humming.

There are five main Yin Organ networks, each paired with a complementary Yang Organ. The Yin Organs take nourishment—the food we eat, the air we breathe, the thoughts going through our minds, the emotions we feel—and transform them into Qi, Blood, and Essence. Yang Organs grasp the debris, the non-nourishing matter, break it down, and excrete it from the body. The five paired Organ networks are:

- Kidneys (Yin) and Bladder (Yang)
- Spleen (Yin) and Stomach (Yang)
- Lungs (Yin) and Large Intestine (Yang)
- Heart (Yin) and Small Intestine (Yang)
- Liver (Yin) and Gallbladder (Yang)

There is also a sixth Organ that works as a channel to protect the Heart. It is called the Pericardium (Yin), which corresponds with its pair, the Triple Heater (Yang).

These Organ networks are what we might refer to as the workhorses of human existence. They are crucial to the sustenance of life. Unlike the organs of anatomical function recognized by Western medicine, each of the Chinese Organs has specific and multiple functions that contribute to our internal health, physical appearance, mental capacity, and personality traits.

When your Organ systems are strong, healthy, and balanced, then you are in good health and your overall appearance is youthful and lustrous. When your Organ systems are weak, unhealthy, and out of balance, then your energy and physical health suffer and manifest as facial concerns, such as wrinkles, loss of muscle tone, and skin problems.

The five Organ networks play a key role in this book because each manages a specific component of our cosmetic appearance, which is driven by their relationship with Qi and Blood:

- The Kidneys store and produce Qi and distribute it to the other Organs. Therefore, they are responsible for the overall vitality and quality of your appearance. They govern the overall aging process.
- The Spleen takes the food and beverages we consume, turns the good nourishment into Essence, and sends it to other Organs. Therefore, the Spleen governs the health, tone, and integrity of the muscles of your face and body.
- The Lungs receive the Essence of food and beverages from the Spleen and mix it with the air your body absorbs to make Qi, then circulate it through the body. Therefore, the Lungs govern the health of skin and the size and integrity of the skin's pores.
- The Heart absorbs Spleen Essence and turns it into Blood and fluids and circulates it through the body. Therefore, it is responsible for the color and the vitality of the complexion.
- The Liver rules the movement and fluidity of Qi and the way Blood flows through the face and body. Therefore, the Liver is responsible for the relaxation and contraction of muscles, tendons, and ligaments, and the way the skin wrinkles.

In Chinese medicine, internal health and physical appearance are measured in terms of the vitality of all the Organs and their ability to function independently and in relation to one another. When you get ill, or your energy is low, or you get dark circles under the eyes, even when you can't think properly, it probably means that there is a disturbance in one or more of your Organs. You have moved from a state of harmony to disharmony. When balance is restored, harmony returns.

Organ Type: Your Strength and Weakness

Though we are made up of all the Organs, each us has a tendency to "favor" a specific Organ, just as we prefer one flavor of ice cream or style of dress over another. This is called your Organ type.

Each Organ contributes a set of characteristics to your existence. Your stature, the quality of your appearance, your personality, and your emotional makeup are all a reflection of your Organ type. So, too, is your susceptibility to illness. When you are in balance and your Qi is flowing smoothly, you personify the strengths of your Organ type. When you are out of balance, the strengths become weaknesses and you fall prey to them. It can have a negative impact on all aspects of your life—your health, your personality, your physical appearance, and your mental stability.

For example, when the Spleen is weak, it shows up in your cosmetic appearance as sagging facial muscles; rather than being nurturing, you might become overbearing. When your Lungs are affected, your skin condition changes and you are susceptible to dry skin or breakouts; interest in life may change to indifference. If your Heart becomes hindered, you are prone to broken capillaries and skin irritation. Your zest for fun and entertainment might wane, and your emotions may fly out of control. Irregularities in your Liver lead to wrinkles, and you may grow angry and intolerant. And if your Kidneys slow down, the aging process accelerates and you might become fearful or withdrawn.

We are all susceptible to imbalances and their consequences in any Organ system. However, we are most vulnerable to the conditions that create disturbances in our Organ type. This is best understood by recognizing the unique patterns associated with each Organ and how they relate to life.

Your Emotional ID

We continuously experience an array of emotions, and we all have a personal way of handling them. When we are in harmony, we have a good grasp on our emotions. When we are out of harmony, we can become emotionally fragile. We each have a dominant emotion to which we are most sensitive, and it is linked to our Organ type:

- Kidneys: Fear
- Spleen: Worry
- Lungs: Grief
- Heart: Joy
- Liver: Anger

This does not mean that Heart types are always happy and Liver types are always annoyed about something. What it means is that our Organ health can be affected by too much or too little of its corresponding emotion. A Kidney type, for example, may be a fraidy cat about entering a dark room at night, but when the Kidneys are hindered, that fear can escalate and even turn into a phobia. Heart types are very even-tempered, but too much joy (excitement), say winning the lottery, can cause them to become frantic, anxious, and spin their Heart right out of harmony.

For anyone, excessive exposure to emotion can cause an imbalance in its associated Organ, and an Organ imbalance can cause excessive emotion. Being aware of your dominant emotion can help keep it in check.

There Is a Time and a Season

You know when you have those good days and bad days? Next time, check the calendar and your watch to see how it corresponds to your Organ type.

Each Organ corresponds to a season. When your Organ is in its season, it is the time of year in which you will feel your best, do your best, and look your best. It is also the season in which your Organ is most vulnerable to getting out of harmony, in which case you can experience the opposite reaction. When your Organ is "in season," it is the time to be most vigilant about your health, diet, lifestyle habits, and taking care of your face. These are the seasons corresponding to each Organ:

- Kidneys—Winter
- Spleen—Between seasons
- Lungs—Fall

- Heart—Summer
- Liver—Spring

By the same token, there are times of the day in which the Chinese Organs are most active. It's why your energy peaks at certain times and you can feel physically and mentally challenged at other times.

Chinese medicine has its own theory about the body clock, which says that Qi has a peak flow time through each Organ that corresponds with the twenty-four-hour cycle. Each peak time lasts for two hours. During this time slot, each Organ dominates physically and emotionally. This means you can feel physical and emotional highs when your Organ type is at its peak and in harmony, or lows if it is out of harmony. You'll notice that an Organ's Yin and Yang times fall within a four-hour period.

3 a.m. to 5 a.m. is Lung (Yin) time. While you are still asleep, your Lungs are recharging to clear the air so you wake up refreshed and glide through the day. If you wake too early or do not wake up with energy, it can be linked to the Lungs' inability to produce or distribute Qi and possibly to its associated emotion, grief, which can also be felt as detachment.

5 a.m. to 7 a.m. is Large Intestine (Yang) time. If your Organs are in harmony, this is the optimum time to be moving your bowels. You should train your gut for morning regularity, as Large Intestine time makes for the most efficient elimination of waste. It's a time for letting go.

7 a.m. to 9 a.m. is Stomach (Yang) time. This is the optimum meal-time and the perfect time of day to have breakfast, because your ability to digest is at its peak. You may have trouble eating and assimilating your food when you are worried, because this emotion is associated with the Stomach's Yin counterpart, the Spleen.

9 a.m. to 11 a.m. is Spleen (Yin) time. This is the time to digest. Chinese medicine considers the Spleen most important to transform and transport vital nutrients from your food and beverages. Digestion problems that rock at this time are caused by emotional turmoil linked to worry or mental exhaustion.

11 a.m. to 1 p.m. is Heart (Yin) time. Because the Heart controls all of the emotions and is linked to joy, this is the time of day when Heart types will feel at their peak. Any physical or emotional problems you experience at this time can be linked to a blockage in your Heart.

1 p.m. to 3 p.m. is Small Intestine (Yang) time. This is the ideal time to have lunch. It is also a time for mental clarity and judgment. If you are feeling confused and unable to sort your feelings from your actions, look at your Small Intestine and your Heart.

3 p.m. to 5 p.m. is Bladder (Yang) time. This is the time when your Bladder should be most active. Any interference in Bladder health can be associated with the inability to sort fluids, which can be caused by fear or foreboding, the emotions linked to the Bladder's Yin counterpart, the Kidneys.

5 p.m. to 7 p.m. is Kidney (Yin) time. This is the time of day when your body and Organs begin to wind down and refuel. The Kidneys, the root of life, are also associated with the root of most feelings, which is fear. At this time fear can be at its height. Fear can also be defined as loss of willpower, loneliness, or a sense of insecurity.

7 p.m. to 9 p.m. is Pericardium (Yin) time. Because the Pericardium is linked to the Heart, it, too, is associated with your emotions. This is a time for enjoying what you love to do.

9 p.m. to 11 p.m. is Triple Heater (Yang) time. This Organ is linked to your ability to filter and discharge unwanted body fluids and emotions. At this time you should be feeling happy with peace of mind to take you to sleep.

11 p.m. to 1 a.m. is Gallbladder (Yang) time. The Gallbladder is linked to wise judgment. Problems with sleep at this hour can be caused by emotional turmoil involving decision making and the inability to speak your mind.

1 a.m. to 3 a.m. is Liver (Yin) time. This is a time for sleep, as Liver Blood is being stored and Qi being regulated. If you are awake, it can mean the Liver is struggling to maintain its balance. It can set off your emotions, namely frustration, resentment, and bitterness. You might find yourself rehashing what didn't go right with your day and what is not going right with your life.

Metaphors of Nature

According to Chinese medicine, each Organ parallels with a seasonal cycle. Chinese medicine refers to this as an Organ's phase or element. These five phases represent the stages of the seasons. All the elements are metaphors for substances in nature.

- Kidneys correspond to winter and are associated with storage.
- Spleen corresponds to the changes of season and is associated with transformation.
- Lungs correspond to fall and are associated with harvest.
- Heart corresponds with summer and is associated with growth.
- Liver corresponds with spring and is associated with birth.

Within the seasonal cycle, each Organ is also assigned an element, or basic quality:

- The Kidney/Bladder Systems are related to the element Water. Water moistens the body then resides in the Kidneys. Kidneys depend on moisture to thrive. Without it they wither—and we age. The movement of Water is downward, symbolizing the Kidneys as the Root of Life, the foundation of all of the other Organs.
- The Spleen/Stomach Systems are related to the element Earth. It is a metaphor for productivity and transformation. Spleen is the nurturer, and it begins the process of turning what we consume into Essence. The energy of the Earth is neutral and hence represents the balance of the other Organs.
- The Lung/Large Intestine Systems are related to the element Metal. It is a metaphor for the Lungs' role as conductor of the movement of Qi throughout the body. The movement of Metal is contractive and inward. Like the Lung personality, it represents this Organ's ability to be molded yet still remain firm.
- The Heart/Small Intestine Systems are related to the element Fire. It is a metaphor for energy created by the Heart. It is why a Heart type is filled with joy and excitement about life. The energy of Fire is upward. It can sparkle or flare.
- The Liver/Gallbladder Systems are related to the element Wood. It is symbolic of strength and stability. Since the energy of Wood is expansive and outward, it can be both strong and pliable.

The Six Evils

Chinese medicine recognizes six climatic interactions that can throw us off our game and knock us out of balance. Referred to as the six "evils," they, too, are metaphors of nature that relate to the weather and the effects it has on our Organs.

In nature, if the temperature gets too cold, plants freeze and die. When it gets too hot, plant life scorches and burns. Excessive dryness causes dehydration and death. As in nature, the havoc caused outside of your body also occurs internally. Any one of the evils can be exacerbated by stress or a poor diet. Lifestyle plays a role as well, and includes excessive sexual activity, sun exposure, alcohol, nicotine, and lack of sleep, to name but a few.

Cold affects the Kidneys and Bladder. If the Kidney Organ lacks warmth, it becomes immobilized. It causes the body to contract and obstructs normal movement. If this system is affected by cold, you may experience premature aging, a pale, puffy face, lethargy, chills, or low back pain.

Dampness affects the Spleen and Stomach. Dampness causes things to become "bogged down." Damp conditions make you feel heavy, foggy, and sluggish. Dampness of the Spleen causes facial and body bloating, sagging muscles, inability to lose weight, digestive problems, and a feeling of heaviness and weakness in your arms and legs.

Dryness affects the Lungs and Large Intestine. Dryness refers to dehydration. Signs of dryness are dry, dull, and lifeless-looking or cracked skin. It can also cause a dry cough, thirst, and constipation.

Heat and Fire are interchangeable and affect the Heart and Small Intestine. They can break capillaries on your cheeks, forehead, and chin, and can cause skin redness, irritation, rashes, even a fever.

Wind affects the Liver and Gallbladder. It is quick, light, and dry and produces change and reckless movement that would otherwise be smooth. If wind is causing your Qi to go awry in your tendons and muscle fibers, they will not be able to contract and relax smoothly, causing wrinkles. Wind can also cause headaches, dizziness, facial tics, or facial spasms.

Orifice: Guarding Health

According to Chinese medicine, the Meridians of each Organ connect to or travel through an orifice. Problems with their associated senses can be a reflection of disharmony within its related Organ. For example, a chronic ear or hearing problem can be due to a Kidney deficiency, mouth and lip problems can be indicative of a Spleen deficiency, and a dry nose can suggest a Lung problem. A red hot tongue can be due to a Heart disturbance, and blurred or irritated eyes can be a manifestation of a problem in the Liver. These are the Organs and their related orifices:

- Kidneys—Ears
- Spleen—Mouth
- Lungs—Nose
- Heart—Tongue
- Liver—Eyes

Food and Your Organs

Asian culture views food differently than the Western world does. In the West, it is the nutrient value of the food that is emphasized—protein, carbohydrate, fat, vitamin, mineral, and fiber content. Eastern medicine, on the other hand, looks at the internal effect on your Organs that is created when a given food is consumed. This is why nourishing your body properly is so intricately tied to your Organs, Qi, your Organ type, and, ultimately, balance—and why you'll be reading a lot about foods and eating right for your Organ type in this book.

Chinese medicine divides foods into their Yin and Yang properties. Eating Yin foods helps your body to become more Yin, and eating Yang foods helps you to become more Yang. For example, if you look puffy and pale and feel tired all over, an Eastern medicine doctor will tell you to eat pork with black beans and shiitake mushrooms—all Yang-producing foods. They will reduce your puffiness, give you color, and boost your energy.

Yin and Yang foods can also produce or dry moisture in the skin of your face and body. If you have dry skin and small pores, the same Chinese practitioner would recommend eating baked tofu with cauliflower and white rice. Tofu, cauliflower, and white rice are moisture-producing Yin foods. When consumed, they will moisten your skin and balance your pores.

Foods not only have moisture-producing properties, but also have a direction of flow. Some foods send their energy inward toward your Organs. Some move their energy outward to the surface of your skin. Some send their energy upward to the top of your head, while others move it downward toward your feet. Peppermint, for example, sends its cooling energy upward toward the surface of your body and cools you down. Cayenne pepper sends its energy inward to help you feel warm.

- Upward-moving foods are good to eat in the spring.
- Outward-moving foods are good to eat in the summer.
- Downward-moving foods are good to eat in the fall.
- Inward-moving foods are good to eat in the winter.

Your Organs have color affiliations with different foods as well. Specific food colors and flavors have beneficial effects on different Organ systems.

The color of a food refers to its visual appearance, but in Chinese medicines it represents *your* visual appearance:

- Yellow is for the Spleen and represents a yellowish cast on your face. Yellow foods include spaghetti squash and sweet potatoes. Spleen yellow also refers to foods with a yellow-orange hue, such as butternut squash and yams.
- White is for the Lungs and is seen as a pale white face. White foods such as potatoes, tofu, and white fish feed the Lungs.
- Red is for the Heart. If your face is red or flushes easily, you may have an imbalance in your Heart. Eat red-colored foods such as beets, red snapper, and red berries.
- Green is for the Liver. A greenish cast on your face may be indicative of a Liver disharmony. In this case, eating foods such as green apples, kiwis, and most green vegetables will help heal the Liver.
- If your face has a black or dark bluish hue, look at your Kidneys. Eating dark-colored foods such as black beans, blueberries, blackberries, and black sesame seeds will nourish and support the Kidneys.

Like the color of a food, the flavor of a food is also connected to the Organs. Some food flavors are easy to determine. Figs and carrots taste sweet. Pepper and curry powder make food taste spicy. Chicory and coffee taste bitter. Lemons and sour plums taste sour. Seaweed and cured olives taste salty.

Other foods, however, have more subtle flavors and their tastes may be more difficult to determine. In this case, the food is categorized according to the time-tested effect that it has on your Organs. For example, kidney beans may not taste particularly sweet, but because they nourish the Spleen, they fall into the sweet category. A bay leaf, although a spice, doesn't taste spicy, but because it has beneficial effects on the Lungs, it is placed in the spicy category. The same is true of papaya. Papaya tastes sweet and helps the heart, so it is considered both a sweet and a bitter food. For the same reason, tomatoes are a sour food for the Liver, and tuna fish is a salty food that helps the Kidneys.

This is how color and flavor relate to each Organ type.

ORGAN	COLOR	FLAVOR
Spleen	Yellow	Sweet
Lungs	White	Spicy
Heart	Red	Bitter
Liver	Green	Sour
Kidneys	Black/Dark Blue	Salty

As you can see, the relationship between Chinese medicine and food—and by extension, your face—is intricate. More information and how to select foods based on your Organ type and beauty goals can be found in Chapter 10.

Meridians: Internal Pathways

Just as a meridian is an imaginary line on the Earth's surface, Meridians in Eastern medicine are pathways in which Qi and Blood travel in constant motion through the body to and from the Organs. Like the Organs, these pathways cannot be seen or felt, but they are not imaginary.

There are twelve bilateral pairs of Meridians that correspond to the

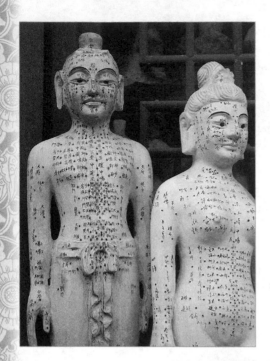

twelve Yin and Yang Organs. They run symmetrically on the right and left sides of the body. Meridians connect to one another and loop around the body in a specific direction. As a Meridian passes through an Organ, it assumes its name and attributes. For instance, as a Meridian passes through the Lung Organ, its name becomes the Lung Meridian. So if the Qi of the Lung Organ is weak, the Qi of the Lung Meridian will also be weak. As you will see later, there are also two additional vessels—the conception vessel that travels up the front of your body, and the governing vessel that traverses the back.

Meridians are the keys to both wellness and preventing disease in Chinese medicine. Acupuncturists place hair-thin sterile needles into sites along the Meridians of specific Organs to get Qi and Blood flowing and get them back into balance. These sites, called acupuncture points, are numbered according to an Organ's pathway, each beginning with the number one. Meridian lengths vary, as does the number of points per pathway. For example, Spleen 6 (SP 6) is the sixth point in the Spleen Meridian, Stomach 36 (ST 36) is the thirty-sixth point in the Stomach Meridian, and Large Intestine 4 (LI 4) is the fourth point on the Large Intestine Meridian.

Above is an illustration of figures showing the flow of Meridians and all of the acupuncture points. There are more than 365 points on the body. In this book, we will be focusing on the forty-six points that apply to cosmetic concerns. The only difference between what I do and what I am going to teach you to do is that you will be using acupressure instead of acupuncture.

Touch and Go: Key Acupressure Points

The principles of acupressure are the same as those of acupuncture. The purpose is to have Qi and Blood move freely through the Meridians and Organs. So manually pressing, holding, or rubbing the points in a specific sequence along a Meridian can move the Qi and Blood when they are stuck, calm them when they are too active, and increase them when they are lacking. Working on your body in this way will help you:

- Eliminate fine lines
- Soften deep wrinkles
- Tone, relax, and nourish muscles
- Improve skin texture, color, and luster
- Increase energy in skin cells and tissue
- Enhance overall appearance and health
- Correct Organ imbalances and deficiencies
- Reduce physical, mental, and emotional stress and tension

A form of acupressure known as Tui Na (pronounced *twee na*) is commonly used throughout Asian countries to treat many health conditions. An integral part of Eastern medicine, it is taught as part of the formal curriculum in Chinese medical training. *Tui na* in Chinese means "push-grasp" or "poke-pinch." Typically it is a series of pressing, tapping, and kneading motions in which you use the palms, fingertips, knuckles, or a special tool to generate energy flow through the Meridians and balance the Organs.

In this book, the type of acupressure that you will be applying is similar to that of Tui Na. Your thumbs and fingertips will do most of the work. No routine will take more than twenty minutes, including the total AcuFacial® Acupressure Facelift. Most of the other treatments, which target specific

---

ALTERNATIVE: ACUPRESSURE TOOL

You can massage acupressure points by using the pad of a finger (usually your index finger). However, if you have arthritic fingers, or your fingers do not exert enough pressure, or if you maintain long fingernails, massaging in this fashion can be problematic.

As an alternative, you can use your knuckle or a special tool designed specifically to move energy. The tool looks like a metal pen and is infused with energy, so it actually adds Qi to your treatment. You can find out more about it on my website, at www.hamptonsacupuncture.com.

Organs and health problems, are shorter. After a day or two of practice, the points will be easy to find and the facelift treatment and other routines you choose will be easy to do.

FEELING THE PRESSURE

Most acupressure points are located in indentations or on top of slight bulges on the surface of the skin. They are easy to locate just by using light pressure. There are also illustrations throughout the book to guide you. You can use your thumb, index, or middle finger to work them. You'll apply medium-to-firm pressure—about the amount of pressure you'd use to shake a hand—for most of the pressure points. When working on the face, you'll want to use slightly less pressure, about the amount you'd use when testing an avocado or melon for ripeness. You will massage each point in a circular motion for ten rotations—and this is *very* important—in a clockwise direction. You will do each section three times as part of the routine.

For the most part, pressure points are located on both sides of the body. Except for your arms, you can massage them simultaneously or one at a time. Pay attention to the direction of your rotations if you are doing both sides of the body at once, as it is the natural tendency for most people to move inward or away from the body when working the fingers in tandem. If it feels awkward to you at first, a little practice should overcome the tendency. Or, although it will take longer, you can simply do the points one at a time.

There are many opportunities throughout the day to give yourself a quick treatment. For instance, you can do acupressure while waiting in a line, taking a bath, or even watching television. It is easy and it is relaxing.

If you do the acupressure properly, you should feel a difference almost immediately; when you

MERIDIAN ABBREVIATIONS

These are the acupressure abbreviations used in this book:

Kidney Meridian	(K)
Bladder Meridian	(BL)
Spleen Meridian	(SP)
Stomach Meridian	(ST)
Lung Meridian	(L)
Large Intestine Meridian	(LI)
Heart Meridian	(HT)
Small Intestine Meridian	(SI)
Liver Meridian	(LV)
Gallbladder Meridian	(GB)
Pericardium Meridian	(P)
Triple Heater Meridian	(TH)
Conception Vessel	(CV)
Governing Vessel	(GV)

practice it daily, you should start noticing a change in the way you look and feel within one week.

Later in the book, I will help you identify your Organ type—a key to understanding your changing face. But first let's get to the heart of the book, the program that you'll be working on for twenty minutes a day for the next twenty days—my AcuFacial® Acupressure Facelift.

3

Getting Your Best Face *Now:* The AcuFacial® Acupressure Facelift

WHO DOESN'T WANT TO LOOK REFRESHED, renewed, and more radiant! Most people, however, can only dream of having access to the same age-defying treatments that give celebrities, socialites, supermodels, and executives their smashing great looks. But now there is a way to achieve that dream.

The AcuFacial® Acupressure Facelift is the noninvasive, easy-to-perform, do-it-yourself, affordable alternative to an expensive facelift, brow lift, Botox treatment, or any of the other surgical treatments aimed at shaving years off your looks. It is a holistic approach that lifts and tones sagging facial muscles back into shape by using the manual version of acupuncture. When facial muscles lift and tone, the skin over them also tightens, easing sagging, out-of-contour skin. Fine lines disappear, deep wrinkles soften, your complexion brightens, and your cheeks, neck, and jawline get more definition. The result is a soft, luminous, youthful glow that you—and others—can't help noticing. It's like taking your face to the gym! By doing the AcuFacial® Acupressure Facelift and following it as prescribed, you'll have people guessing what you've "had done" to make you look so good.

As stated before, the AcuFacial® Acupressure Facelift is based on the ancient Chinese style of acupressure called Tui Na (pronounced *twee-na*), in which you manually press and knead the same key points I use to give an acupuncture facelift to my clients. You'll use the pads of your fingertips to do the same work on sites located in indentations, or slight bulges, on the skin of the feet, legs, hands, arms, neck, face, and head. It is easy and relaxing, and can be done just about anywhere.

The AcuFacial® Acupressure Facelift involves thirty-eight specific sites and takes about twenty minutes a day. Do it every day for twenty days, and I promise you'll see a noticeable difference. The more you do it, the better you'll look. You'll reap the best rewards if you also follow the dietary advice for your Organ type and the skin care recommendations you'll find in Chapter 10. For specific cosmetic problems, you can follow the protocols recommended in any of the Organ chapters to give you extra help. However, if you do nothing but the AcuFacial® Acupressure Facelift, you'll still get noticeable, rejuvenating results.

Though you can do the facelift anywhere and at any time, I find the best time to perform it is before going to bed at night or when you first get up in the morning. For one, it is relaxing. You'll also most likely be wearing loose clothing, which will allow you to access the points more easily. You can do acupressure on top of clothing (as long as you can feel the effect), but it is best to apply pressure directly to the skin.

The facelift starts at the feet and works its way to the face and head. You'll apply moderate to firm pressure to the key points in a circular motion for ten rotations in a clockwise direction. Once you're done, you'll have massaged each point three times. Before getting started, make sure to read "Touch and Go: Key Acupressure Points" (see page 30), which teaches you the nuances of performing acupressure effectively. You may also want to browse the appendix for more information on the benefits of each point.

Applying pressure in this fashion to key Meridians on the body will have an immediate impact. As you've learned in this book, acupressure corrects imbalances in the body's Organ systems. When Qi is stuck, flows too swiftly, or flows erratically, it negatively affects your internal health, which shows up externally as unflattering visible signs of aging. This doesn't have to be. When your Organs are working at their best, you feel your best and look your best.

The AcuFacial® Acupressure Facelift, as well as the other treatments featured in this book, is not only curative—but also preventive. And it's never too late to start. However, doing this technique before lines and wrinkles start to appear can hold them off for years to come. It's possible you may never look your chronological age! The AcuFacial® Acupressure Facelift works because it:

- Tones sagging facial muscles, jowls, and frown lines
- Eliminates fine lines
- Diminishes wrinkles and creases across the forehead, between the eyebrows, and around the eyes
- Reduces undereye and face puffiness
- Reduces large and uneven facial pores
- Firms and improves skin quality and texture
- Gives the face a luminous and radiant glow

In addition, the AcuFacial® Acupressure Facelift helps achieve better health. You'll feel better because it:

- Reduces stress
- Encourages overall health
- Eliminates fatigue
- Improves circulation
- Stimulates lymphatic drainage
- Induces relaxation
- Strengthens the immune system
- Increases energy and promotes a sense of well-being
- Produces more restful sleep
- Improves concentration and mental clarity
- Gives you a greater sense of contentment

Now, let's get started.

> **NOTE:** If you are pregnant, or think you may be, be sure to consult your physician before starting this program. In addition, *avoid* the following acupressure points: LV 3, SP 6, SP 10, and LI 4.

AcuFacial® Acupressure Facelift

The facelift begins and ends with one point on the face called Yin Tang, which will help relax your face and body. It continues with key acupressure points on the feet, then moves to the ankles, legs, wrists, hands, elbows, the back of the neck, and then the face and head. If you find that the entire regime takes more than twenty minutes, you can exchange points LV 3, K 3, and SP 3 and point SP 6. See page 231 for the proper location.

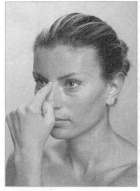

Yin Tang

FACE

Do ten clockwise rotations before moving on.

Yin Tang | This is an extra point, meaning it's not on an Organ Meridian. This point is located between your eyebrows and above the nose. In addition to relaxing your face and body, it softens and helps prevent wrinkles between the eyebrows.

FEET AND LEGS

Do ten rotations of each point on both feet and legs, one at a time or simultaneously. Repeat the sequence two more times before moving on.

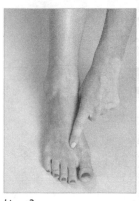

Liver 3

Liver 3 | Slide your finger between your big toe and second toe on the top of your foot. When you reach the intersection of the first and second toes, you are on LV 3. This point softens wrinkles, lightens sunspots, and calms eye twitches and muscle spasms. It also helps clear acne and pimples.

Spleen 3 | SP 3 is located on the inside of your foot, below the base of the large toe, on the edge of the dark and light skin. This point lifts sagging cheek muscles and strengthens the Spleen.

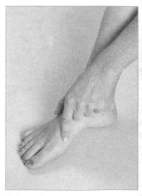

Spleen 3

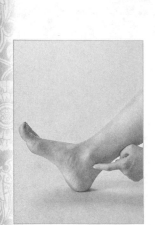

Kidney 3

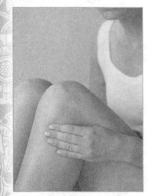

Stomach 36 (a)

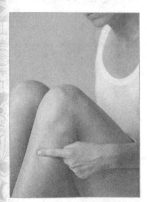

Stomach 36 (b)

Kidney 3 | K 3 is located in the soft spot on the inside of your ankle, between the inside ankle bone and the tendon. This point decreases facial swelling and strengthens the Kidneys.

Stomach 36 | Now we move to the knees. ST 36 is located on the outside of the leg below the knee. It is found in the depression approximately four finger-widths below the outside of the leg bone, or fibula. This point helps lift cheek muscles.

Gallbladder 34 | GB 34 is located below the outside of your knee, at the head of the fibula. This point relaxes the Liver and the forehead.

Bladder 40 | BL 40 is located in the back of your knee between the two tendons. This point relaxes the head and forehead.

Spleen 10 | Move to the top of your knees on the inside of your legs. Bend one knee and place the palm of your opposite hand around your knee with the thumb extended upward. Your thumb should fall on a depression above the knee on the inside of the leg. This is SP 10. This point, when combined with LV 3 and LI 11, lightens sunspots.

HANDS AND ARMS

Do ten rotations of each point on both hands and arms. Repeat the sequence two more times before moving on.

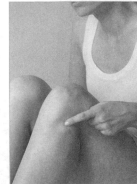

Gallbladder 34

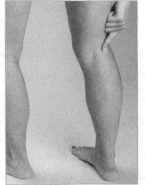

Bladder 40

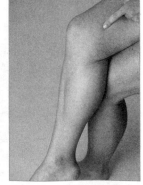

Spleen 10

Lung 9 | Here we start at the wrist. Bend your wrist forward toward your inner arm. L 9 is located on the indentation of your wrist, below your thumb and between the thumb bone and the tendon. Relax your hand before doing the massage. This point helps reduce facial puffiness.

Heart 7 | Still on the wrist, move your finger across and directly below the little finger. HT 7 is in the indentation next to the tendon. This point helps relieve redness in the face, relax the face, and calm the Heart.

Large Intestine 4 | Hold your hand straight up with fingers and thumb together. LI 4 is on the back of the hand, on the soft spot at the bottom of the crease between the thumb and index finger. This point sends Qi to the face. It lifts and tones facial muscles, and helps repair any face or face-related concerns.

Large Intestine 11 | Bend your elbow in front of you at a 90-degree angle. You'll find LI 11 in the indentation on the outside edge of the elbow crease. This point tones facial muscles. It also reduces the redness of pimples and acne. When combined with LV 3 and SP 10 it lightens sunspots.

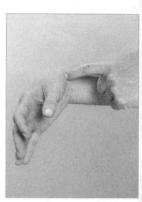

Lung 9

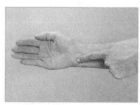

Heart 7

NECK

Do ten rotations of each point. Repeat the sequence two more times before moving on.

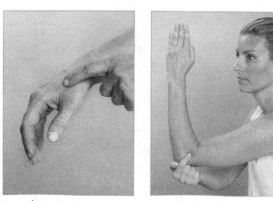

Large Intestine 4   *Large Intestine 11*

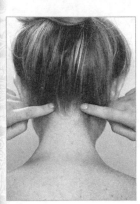

Bladder 10

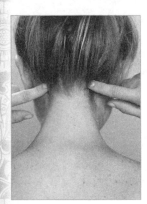

Gallbladder 20

Bladder 10 | Move both hands to the back of your neck and place your fingers in the center of your spine, below the base of the skull. Slide your hands toward your ears until you land in a notch approximately one finger-width away from the center. BL 10 opens the back of the neck to increase the flow of Qi and Blood to the head.

Gallbladder 20 | From BL 10, slide your hands another finger-width toward your ears. The indentation here is GB 20. Like BL 10, it opens up the back of the neck to increase the flow of Qi and Blood to the head. It also reduces wrinkles around the eyes and forehead, and relaxes muscle tension.

Triple Heater 17 | Now, slide your fingers toward your ears. You'll find TH 17 behind the sternocleidomastoid (SCM), the long muscle extending from your jaw to your collarbone, in the depression below your ears at the base of the skull. This point reduces facial puffiness and improves lymph drainage.

Small Intestine 17 | From TH 17, slide your fingers in front of the SCM. This is SI 17, used to relax neck muscles and tighten skin.

Conception Vessel 23 | Move one hand to the front of the neck. CV 23 is found above the Adam's apple and at the base of the chin parallel to the center of the chin. This point lifts muscles in the neck and chin.

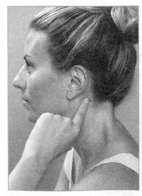

Triple Heater 17

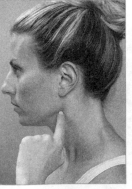

Small Intestine 17

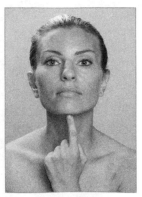

Conception Vessel 23

HEAD

Do ten rotations of each point, then repeat the sequence two more times before moving on.

Conception Vessel 24 | Slide your finger up over your chin to the indentation in the center of your chin, below the lower lip at the base of the gum. This is CV 24. It lifts all the muscles of the face, particularly those around the mouth. It also helps reduce facial puffiness.

Governing Vessel 26 | GV 26 is centrally located between the tip of your nose and the top of your lip. It lifts the muscles of your face and sharpens the mind.

Governing Vessel 20 | GV 20 is located on the top of the head. You can find it by placing your thumbs on your skull at the top of your ears and your fingers on the top of your head. The point is where the middle fingers meet. It lifts facial muscles and clears the mind.

LOWER CHEEK AND JAWLINE

Do ten rotations of each of the next six points, then repeat the sequence two more times before moving on.

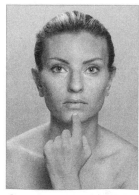

Conception Vessel 24

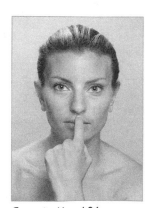

Governing Vessel 26

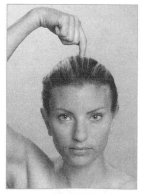

Governing Vessel 20

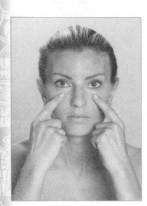

Stomach 2

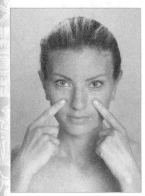

Stomach 3

Stomach 2 | ST 2 is located below the center of the eyes below the bone surrounding the eye. In sequence with the next five points below, it lifts the cheek muscles.

Stomach 3 | ST 3 is located directly below the center of the eyes at the level of the nostrils. It lifts cheek muscles and helps eliminate the nasolabial fold, the creases that extend from the base of the nose to the mouth. It also relieves sinus problems and congestion.

Stomach 4 | Move your finger down close to the corners of your mouth. This is ST 4. It lifts and tones sagging cheek muscles and helps reduce the nasolabial fold.

Stomach 5 | ST 5 is located above the jawline, one finger-width in front of ST 6. With ST 4 and ST 6 it relaxes the jaw and tightens the jawline.

Stomach 6 | Now, move your fingers out toward the jaw joint. ST 6 is located one finger-width above and behind the angle of the jaw. This point lifts cheek and jaw muscles.

Stomach 7 | Now move to the front of your ears. You can find ST 7 by feeling for the depression between the cheekbone and the jawbone. You can feel it move if you open and close your mouth. This points lifts the cheek muscles.

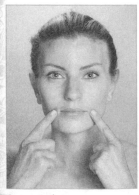

Stomach 4

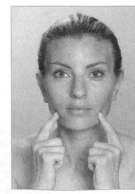

Stomach 5

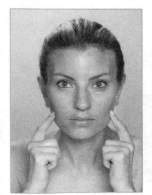

Stomach 6

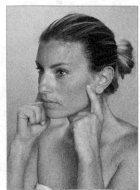

Stomach 7

UPPER CHEEK

Do ten rotations of the next five acupressure points, then repeat the sequence two more times before moving on.

Large Intestine 19 | LI 19 is located between the nostrils and upper lip on either side of GV 26. It reduces wrinkles above the lips.

Large Intestine 20 | Now move to the nostrils. LI 20 is located on the depression at the sides of the nostrils. It helps lift the cheek muscles and reduce the nasolabial fold.

Small Intestine 18 | Move your fingers out toward your cheeks. SI 18 is found parallel to LI 20 and directly below the outer edge of the eyes. It tones sagging cheek muscles.

Stomach 7 | You can find ST 7 by feeling for the depression between the cheekbone and the jawbone. You can feel it move if you open and close your mouth. This point lifts cheek muscles.

Stomach 8 | ST 8 is located at the edge of the forehead at the temple, where the hairline begins to turn downward. It lifts the muscles of the cheeks and the forehead.

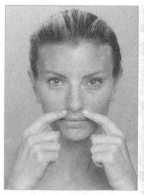

Large Intestine 19

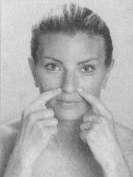

Large Intestine 20

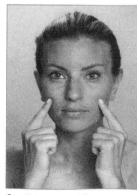

Small Intestine 18

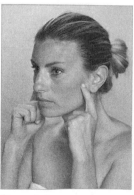

Stomach 7

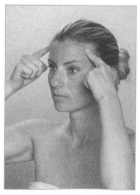

Stomach 8

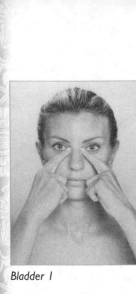

Bladder 1

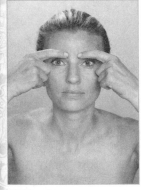

Bladder 2

EYES

Do ten rotations of each of the next five points, then repeat the sequence two more times before moving on.

Bladder 1 | BL 1 is located in the inside corner of your eye, on the side of the nose. It is used for all eye problems.

Bladder 2 | BL 2 is located at the inside edge of your eyebrows, above the inside corner of your eyes. It reduces creases between the eyebrows and forehead.

Yu Yao | This is an extra point, meaning it's not on an Organ Meridian. It is located in the middle of the eyebrow. It softens wrinkles between the eyebrows and across the forehead. It is also used for tension and pain around the eyes.

Gallbladder 1 | GB 1 is located on the outside corner of the eyes. It softens crow's feet around the eyes. With GB 20 and GB 14, it helps alleviate pain located on the side of the head and across the forehead.

Stomach 2 | ST 2 is located below the center of the eyes, under the bone surrounding the eye. In sequence with the points below, it tones the eye muscles.

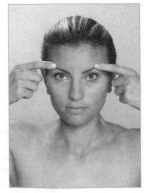

Yu Yao

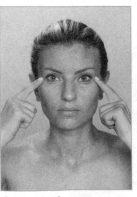

Gallbladder 1

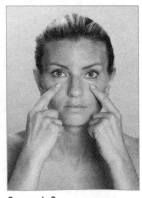

Stomach 2

FOREHEAD

Do ten rotations of each point, then repeat the sequence two more times before moving on.

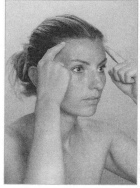

Gallbladder 13

Gallbladder 13 | Divide your hairline as if you had a center part. Follow your hairline from the front center approximately three finger-widths across the hairline. This is GB 13. This point is used for forehead wrinkles.

Gallbladder 14 | GB 14 is located on your forehead, one finger-width above the center of the eyebrow. This is a primary point for wrinkles between the eyes and across the forehead. It is also used to relieve headaches.

Gallbladder 15 | GB 15 is located directly above GB 14 in the hairline. It softens wrinkles and creases across the forehead. It is also used to relieve headaches.

Governing Vessel 20 | Go back to GV 20, which is located on the top of the head. You can find it again by placing your thumbs on your skull at the top of your ears and your fingers on the top of your head. The point is where the middle fingers meet. It is used to lift energy to the top of the head.

FACE

Rotate ten times.

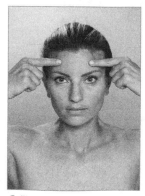

Gallbladder 14

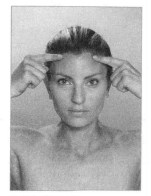

Gallbladder 15

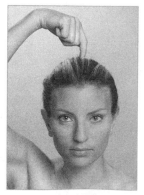

Governing Vessel 20

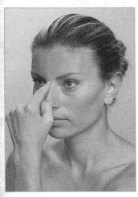

Yin Tang

Yin Tang | Finally, go back to this pressure point on the forehead to finish and relax the face and body.

ACUFACIAL® ACUPRESSURE FACELIFT CHEAT SHEET

After doing the facelift routine a few times, you'll get familiar with the Meridian points and their sites fairly quickly, but it is difficult to remember the order because there are so many! So use this as your cheat sheet. Make a copy of it and keep it at hand wherever you do the routine.

Face	TH 17	ST 7
Yin Tang (10 rotations)	SI 17	ST 8 (3X)
	CV 23 (3X)	
Feet and Legs		**Eyes**
LV 3	**Head**	BL 1
SP 3	CV 24	Yu Yao
K 3	GV 26	BL 2
ST 36	GV 20 (3X)	GB 1
GB 34		ST 2 (3X)
BL 40	**Lower Cheek and Jawline**	
SP 10 (3X)	ST 2	**Forehead**
	ST 3	GB 13
Hands and Arms	ST 4	GB 14
L 9	ST 5	GB 15
H 7	ST 6	GV 20
LI 4	ST 7 (3X)	
LI 11 (3X)		**Face**
	Upper Cheek	Yin Tang (10 rotations)
Neck	LI 19	
BL 10	LI 20	
GB 20	SI 18	

If you are interested in learning more about face muscles—their names, functions, and corresponding acupressure meridians and points, you can find an informative AcuFacial® Muscle Meridian chart on my website: hamptonsacupuncture.com.

4

What's Your Organ Type? Making Your Own Diagnosis

YOU'VE HEARD IT HUNDREDS, PERHAPS EVEN thousands of times: *We all have our strengths and our weaknesses*—a saying that is no more truly expressed than in Chinese medicine. Your Organ type is the Organ that most readily identifies *you*—your state of health, your physical appearance, your personality and emotional makeup, and your spiritual self. Within each, we have our strengths and weaknesses, making these traits, in essence, one and the same—your Organ type.

Your Organ type represents the Organ system to which you are most susceptible in terms of its strengths and weaknesses. This Organ is your asset when it is in balance and your shortcoming when you are off. Discovering your Organ type does not mean there's something wrong with you. In fact, it can be quite the opposite.

You are made up of all of the Organs, and you rely on them at different times. In combination they constitute the ebb and flow of your energetic being. The Liver system kicks in when you need to take action. Rest and renewal relies on the support of your Kidneys. When you are enjoying the achievements and pleasures of life, your Heart is most active. When it is time to analyze, let go, and move on, you call on the Qi of your Lungs. When life throws you a curveball and you stray from your path, it is your Spleen energy that realigns you. So knowing your Organ type, or the Organ system that most reflects your personality, helps you grasp your potential and familiarize yourself with your personal strengths and your potential weaknesses.

When traveling in a group, whether it be friends, colleagues, or even strangers, people automatically assume different roles. Liver types take charge. Heart types entertain. Kidney types sit back and watch. Spleen types keep peace, and you can bet that the Lung types are following the directions or studying the map. Their internal Organ Qi is driving them all, and when they all work cooperatively, it is a peaceful and harmonious journey. By the same token, when your own Organ disharmony prevails, it causes internal chaos and your Organ weakness manifests in an assortment of physical symptoms, including wrinkles and other signs of time you wear on your face.

Knowing your Organ type is your key to correcting the internal condition that shows up as specific signs of aging on your face and in your body; it also helps you recognize who you are, and can be a great tool to help you manage the subtleties of your life.

In a perfect world, everyone would live in a constant state of balance, but that is not realistic. The truth is, the vagaries of life are constantly making you act when you want rest, sleep when you're not tired, or any number of other things that put friction in life. Often it can cause you to forget to enjoy those precious moments, ignore the warning signs of strife, and not only stray from your path but sometimes miss your way completely. There are good days, bad days, and then there are those disastrous days when it seems like your world is in complete disarray. If your Organs are strong and resilient, you are able to deal with the chaos and get back on track with minimal repercussions. If your Organs are weak or lacking, however, it is likely that you will trip, fall, skin your knee, or even find yourself lost in Alice in Wonderland's rabbit hole.

Anything can impact the health of your Organs—your daily activities, mood, diet, physical trauma, the stress of losing a job, the loss of a loved one. The effects show up on your face, and the condition of your facial muscles, skin, and complexion is the primary clue. As you will learn as you read on, the quality of the way you age is related to your Kidneys, the health of your muscles is dominated by your Spleen, the condition of your skin is controlled by your Lungs, the integrity of your capillaries and vessels is a product of your Heart, and muscle movement and Blood flow are driven by your Liver. The key to attaining optimal health is knowing when your Organs are working in harmony, the warning signs of when they are not, and how to correct them before the problems escalate.

The Organ Type Questionnaire

Figuring out your Organ type is relatively easy with this questionnaire. Your answers will pinpoint your Organ type in your current state of health. Since every Organ affects another, you will recognize a little bit of yourself in each, but generally one dominates.

Each grouping that follows contains twenty questions. Answer each question with a *yes* or a *no*. If you answer *yes* to ten or more of the twenty questions in each grouping, you have your diagnosis. If you answer *yes* to ten or more of the questions in more than one Organ, either choose the Organ with the most *yes* answers or read the chapters pertaining to those Organs and see which one resonates the most with you. If you have fewer than ten *yes* answers in all categories, then choose the Organ with the highest number of *yes* answers.

As you will learn, the health of the Kidneys influences all of the Organs, so if you have a lot of *yes* answers in all of the categories, you are probably a Kidney type. If after answering the questions, you are still unsure about your Organ type, repeat the questionnaire with a friend who knows you well. Self-perceptions often differ from the way others perceive you. A trusted friend should be able to help you pinpoint your Organ type.

KIDNEY TYPE

1. Do you have a high forehead, large ears, deep-set eyes, and strong facial features?
2. Do you have premature aging?
3. Do you have early-onset graying, thinning, or balding hair?
4. Do you have puffiness or dark circles under your eyes?
5. Does your face look pale and puffy?
6. Do you have chronic dental problems?

7. Do you have ringing in your ears, difficulty hearing, or hearing loss?
8. Do you have a poor memory?
9. Do you have chronic knee or lower back pain?
10. Do you have porous or brittle bones?
11. Do you tire easily?
12. Did you mature late in life?
13. Do you dislike cold weather?
14. Are you strong-willed and self-sufficient?
15. Do you crave frequent periods of privacy and introspection?
16. Do you often feel withdrawn, depressed, apathetic, or reclusive?
17. Do you easily become frightened, scared, or fearful?
18. Do you see yourself as a philosophizer or truth seeker?
19. Have you lost your spiritual connection?
20. Do you crave salty foods or add extra salt to your meals?

SPLEEN TYPE

1. Do you have strong, thick facial muscles and a round, full figure?
2. Do you have creases around your mouth and a sagging neck or jawline?
3. Does your skin break out under your chin and/or around your mouth?
4. Do you have a pale or yellowish complexion, or a yellowish cast around your mouth?
5. Do you have chronic allergies and sinus congestion?
6. Do you gain weight easily and have difficulty losing it?
7. Do you have frequent indigestion, gas, or bloating, especially after meals?
8. Do you have cellulite?
9. Do you frequently feel tired, heavy, or lethargic?
10. Do you bruise easily?
11. Do you have heaviness or sagging muscles in your abdomen, upper arms, or thighs?
12. Are you down to earth, friendly, and nurturing?
13. Do you see yourself as a mediator, people pleaser, or peacemaker?
14. Do you have difficulty saying no to others?
15. Do you put the needs of others first, to the detriment of your own?
16. Are you a chronic worrier?
17. Do you get flustered and upset when having to compete with others?

18. Do you feel stuck or trapped in your life?
19. Do you crave stability in your life and get upset when it is not status quo?
20. Do you frequently crave sweet or starchy foods?

LUNG TYPE

1. Are you small-boned and angular with soft, prominent features and small, trim, compact muscles?
2. Do you have a pale complexion?
3. Are you prone to oily or dry skin?
4. Are you prone to acne or frequent skin problems?
5. Do you have chronic nasal dryness or sinus congestion?
6. Do you have thin or patchy facial hair, or more body hair than normal?
7. Do you have eczema, psoriasis, or rosacea or frequently break out in a rash?
8. Are you prone to dry coughs or chest congestion?
9. Do you have breathing difficulties, such as shortness of breath or asthma?
10. Do you have a weak voice or do others having difficulty hearing you?
11. Do you get sick easily, particularly in the late fall or early winter?
12. Do you have frequent constipation or bowel problems?
13. Do you observe, study, and analyze situations before acting on them?
14. Are you critical of new situations or other people?
15. Do you enjoy projects that require an analytical, logical, and systematic approach to problem solving?
16. Do you obey rules and work easily in situations where the guidelines and goals are well defined?
17. Are you organized, neat, and orderly?
18. Do you get overwhelmed by your emotions or have difficulty expressing your feelings?
19. Do you need space and prefer spending time alone?
20. Do you often feel sad or forlorn?

HEART TYPE

1. Do you have a sleek and willowy physique?
2. Do you have a long neck and long limbs?

3. Do you have broken capillaries on your face?

4. Do you have patches of red or irritated skin on your face or body?

5. Do you have a pale complexion with fines lines or shallow wrinkles?

6. Is your skin sensitive or reactive?

7. Do you frequently feel flushed or overheated?

8. Do you perspire easily?

9. Do your fingers and hands frequently get swollen or cold?

10. Do you suffer from insomnia, have vivid dreams, or disturbed sleep?

11. Do you have low or high blood pressure?

12. Do you have heart palpitations or heart problems?

13. Do you have poor circulation?

14. Do you like being the "life of the party"?

15. Do you enjoy physical contact and intimacy?

16. Are you intuitive and easily know what others are thinking?

17. Is it easy for you to become restless or anxious?

18. Do you stutter, talk too fast, or giggle when you are nervous?

19. Is it easy for you to get excited or nervous?

20. Do you have frequent mood swings or feel emotionally fragile?

LIVER TYPE

1. Do you have thick, firm skin and solid, robust muscle tone?

2. Do you have wrinkles between your eyebrows, around your eyes, or across your forehead?

3. Do you have irritated or red, itchy eyes (not related to an allergy)?

4. Do you have eye problems, such as spasms, tics, or weak vision?

5. Do you have brownish-colored sunspots or other skin discoloration?

6. Do you frequently get headaches or feel dizzy?

7. Do you frequently get heartburn, acid reflux, or indigestion?

8. Do you frequently feel a knot in your throat or tightness in your chest?

9. Do you have chronic neck or shoulder pain?

10. Are you prone to sciatica, spasms, or nerve pain?

11. Do you have dry, brittle nails?

12. Does windy weather irritate you?

13. Are you competitive?

14. Do you crave action, adventure, and a challenge?

15. Are you confident and assertive?

16. Do you like leading and directing others?

17. Are you comfortable and productive when under pressure?

18. Are you easily affected by stressful situations?

19. Are you easily frustrated, angered, or enraged?

20. Do you often feel impulsive or intolerant?

What to Do with Your Results

Knowing your Organ type does not require self-analysis. It is not better or worse to be one type instead of another. Knowing your type will, however, help you to better understand your state of health and provide insight into the cosmetic changes you are experiencing or may experience at some point in life.

If you would like to learn more about the Organs and your type in particular, the next five chapters are each focused on an individual Organ. Reading about your Organ type will help clarify your answers to the questionnaire. Included in each chapter is one or more acupressure treatments addressing the cosmetic issues that typically dominate that Organ type. You'll also find the diet that's best for each Organ type, plus skin care tips. Following the recommendations for your Organ type will help you keep your Organ in balance. It will also help you enhance the benefits of the natural facelift protocol that is the focus of the book.

It is not necessary to focus separately on the cosmetic issues associated with your Organ type, if you do not desire to do so, because most are already incorporated in the AcuFacial® Acupressure Facelift. If your primary interest is toning your face and looking better than ever, then just stick with the facelift. But if you really want to make a change in your complexion and health, and your *life*, follow the facelift protocol *and* follow the advice in the chapter devoted to your Organ type, plus the other dietary and skin care advice in Chapters 10 and 11.

Before embarking on any treatment, you need to read the section "Touch and Go: Key Acupressure Points" (see page 30), which will help you become expert at performing the acupressure techniques offered in this book.

5

Puffy All Over: Welcome to Your Kidneys

I BEGAN SEEING FRAN TWO MONTHS BEFORE HER fiftieth birthday and three weeks after the death of her mother. Fran had been the primary caretaker for her ninety-eight-year-old mother during a long and lingering illness, so it was no surprise that Fran showed up in my office feeling worn and looking older than her years. Along with everything else going on in her life, what she saw when she looked in the mirror really had her down.

Through most of her adult life, Fran took pride in the way she looked and people often remarked about her youthful appearance and energy. She credited it all to her good genes and positive outlook on life. The compliments, however, were a thing of the past, and she could see why. She looked tired, pale, and puffy. Her dewy skin, which was once the envy of others, looked withered. Her once prominently sculpted high cheekbones were no longer obvious, and her thick, dark hair was drab.

"My hair is actually thinning," she lamented. "Is this really possible for someone my age?" she asked. "Yes," I told her, "but not for the reason that you might be thinking."

I sensed there was more to Fran's mental anguish than the death of her mother. She talked a long time about her mother's slow decline before she got to what else was on her mind. "My memory seems shot," she said. "I try to tell myself I forget to do things because I'm tired, but honestly I'm worried that the same thing is happening to me as happened to my mother. And I'm only fifty years old!"

I smiled at her reassuringly. "I wouldn't jump to too many conclusions," I said. "Let's do some acupuncture so we can get those cheekbones high and showing and see what it does to your outlook on life."

The magnitude of the stress Fran had recently been through could take its toll on anyone's Kidneys, but for a Kidney type like Fran, it can be truly profound.

Profile of a Kidney Type

A Kidney type is probably the easiest to spot by facial features alone. High forehead, sculpted facial features, and deep-set eyes, like Fran's—or, more to the point, what Fran badly desired to reclaim—are characteristic of healthy Kidney types. Also, they typically have thick hair, strong teeth and bones, large earlobes, a sturdy frame, and a fit, dense physique. However, what makes you a Kidney type has a lot more to do with what's going on in your head rather than what you see on the outside.

Kidney types tend to be cerebral. They are the philosophers of the world, strongly rooted and inwardly focused. Both introspective and articulate, they ponder the unknown and express the profound. Healthy Kidney personalities are strong willed, self-sufficient, sharp witted, and ambitious. When Kidney types are out of balance, look out. The change can be remarkable. They can become withdrawn, stubborn, depressed, fearful, apathetic, reclusive, and, like Fran, they will start obsessing about the meaning of life.

As drastically as their personality can change, their physical changes can be even more pro-

> ### SNAPSHOT OF THE
> ### KIDNEYS
>
> *Element:* Water
> *Complementary Organ:* Bladder
> *Primary function:* Regulating the aging process
> *Facial concern:* Premature aging, hair loss
> *Emotional regulation:* Fear
> *Complementary orifice:* Ear
> *Season:* Winter
> *Color:* Black
> *Taste:* Salty
> *Primary evil:* Cold
> *Active time:* 3 p.m. to 7 p.m.

nounced. When the Kidneys are compromised and not corrected, it shows. The face gets puffy or withered, with wrinkles all over, and dark circles form under the eyes, causing a rapidly aging appearance. Hair becomes thin and prematurely gray. Baldness can also develop.

Damage to the Kidneys also takes a toll on your health. If you are genetically prone to weak Kidneys or if you had a severe illness early in life, the physical or emotional trauma can tax your Kidneys. This can cause a delay in physical development, what is often referred to as being a late bloomer. Kidney types may not develop physically, mentally, or sexually until later in life. For young girls and boys, this means a delay in growth and puberty. If your Kidneys are affected during your adult years, signs of aging will start to show prematurely. This means that you will probably look and feel older than other people the same age.

Weak Kidney types are also plagued with chronic lower back, knee, and other bone-related health problems, such as tooth decay, bone fragility, and osteoporosis. Because the orifice associated with the Kidneys is the ear, hearing problems such as poor hearing, hearing loss, and low-pitched ringing in the ears, are associated with the Kidneys. Out-of-balance Kidney types also tend to have poor memory and fatigue easily.

When you put it all together, chronically poor Kidney function can make you feel like you're falling apart, just like Fran. And for good reason. The Kidneys are intrinsically involved in the aging process.

The Role of the Kidneys: Healthy Aging

Eastern and Western medicine view the aging process very differently. According to Western thought, aging occurs when your body's building blocks—your cells—die faster than your body can replace them. There are many reasons why cells die, but the prominent theory is known as oxidation.

When your cells get damaged or old, they wither and die. They also produce substances called free radicals that swarm cells like the little gobblers in the electronic game Pac-Man, invading them and eating everything in sight. As free radicals accumulate, they attack and kill cells faster and faster. The more cells that die, the more difficult it becomes for your body to replace them with new, healthy ones. At some point the scale tips and you begin to lose cells faster than you can make new ones. When this happens, your skin, muscles, and body tissue begin to break down. You start looking old.

Eastern medicine takes a different point of view. Chinese doctors say that aging is not caused by the deterioration of your cells but by the breakdown of your Kidney energy. The Kidneys are known as the Root of Life because they are the core of your existence, as essential to life as a foundation is to a house. If you don't maintain the foundation of your life, it will eventually decay and fall apart. Without healthy Kidneys, you'll mature and age poorly.

The Kidneys sustain the growth and development of your body from birth to death. Healthy Kidneys are vital for proper development during your primary years, your reproductive capability, and the integrity of your body and mind throughout your lifetime, especially in your later years. They are necessary for healthy brain function, strong bones, a thick head of hair, and the fitness of your constitution. Just as the process of birth and growth is determined by the health of your Kidney energy, the process of aging is governed by the weakening of your Kidney energy.

Though you can't live forever, you can delay the signs of aging and ease the physical and mental decline associated with aging by keeping your Kidneys healthy. Fran came from a family with strong Kidney Qi. Her father lived until the age of ninety-five and her mother lived until she was ninety-eight. Her mother was in remarkable health and living on her own until her final year. Up until then, she volunteered at a senior citizens' home, participated in Pilates classes, and took daily walks with her younger friends. Her mind was lucid, sharp, and witty. She knew the names of her local grocer, butcher, and mailman. To top it off, she was also the one who could remember where everybody else had left their keys. Western doctors would attribute a great deal of this to good genes. Eastern doctors would attribute it to strong Kidney energy.

Her decline began with a bout of winter pneumonia. Fran naturally assumed that her mom would bounce back, but she didn't. Watching her mother deteriorate was agonizing for Fran, and realizing the effects that it had on herself at such a young age "frightened her to death."

The Root of Life: How the Kidneys Function

The fact that the Kidneys take such a toll on your health and physical appearance when they are out of harmony indicates their importance to life itself. Your Kidneys are the most vital of all of the Organs. If your Organs were designed to create a car rather than form human existence, the Kidneys would be the engine. Life wouldn't be much good without them. Without Kidney energy, life itself would cease.

Eastern medical doctrine says the Kidneys possess a special kind of Qi, known as Jing. This, like your genes, is what you inherit from your parents and ancestors. Passed down from generation to generation, it is collected, combined with what we eat and drink, and stored in your Kidneys. Jing, Kidney Qi, and Blood are the fuel for the fire that ignites other Organs to do their job.

The Kidneys are responsible for keeping Qi and Blood flowing to all the Organs in a continuum. Although each Organ has its own special function, they are all dependent on the health of the Kidneys to perform their job optimally. The Kidneys are responsible for sending life's essentials, Qi and Blood, to the Spleen. The Spleen takes the foods and beverages that you consume and starts the process of creating Qi by sending a substance called Essence to the Lungs. The Lungs make the Qi and send it down to the Kidneys. The ability for the Lungs to distribute Qi to other Organs and throughout the body is dependent upon the Kidneys' ability to "grasp" the Qi and pull it down from your Lungs. When you can't catch your breath, or as in the type of asthma in which your breathing is worse when you try to inhale, it is because your Kidneys are weak and can't grab and hold on to your Lung Qi. Think of your Lung Qi as an air balloon. If the Kidney Qi is not strong enough to hold on to it, it floats away.

The Kidneys take Lung Qi and separate it into pure Qi—what the body can use—and impure Qi—what the body no longer needs. The pure Qi gets distributed to other Organs and throughout the body. The Kidneys take the impure Qi and send it to their paired Organ, the Bladder, where it gets filtered out of the body as urine.

If your Kidneys are weak, they can't filter properly. What should go down goes up and what should go up goes down. Water accumulates in your face and body. A puffy face, swelling around your eyes, circles below them,

> ## FUNCTIONS OF THE KIDNEYS
>
> The Kidneys team up with the Bladder to:
>
> - Store Essence
> - Produce Marrow for the brain and the bones
> - Oversee the integrity of Qi and Blood for all Organ systems
> - Regulate the aging process
> - Influence mental willpower
> - Keep the hair on your head healthy and strong
> - Control the emotion of fear

and water retention elsewhere in your body are all the result of the Kidneys' inability to filter properly. If the Kidneys are weak, it affects your Bladder and your ability to urinate properly is compromised. This often results in urinary problems, such as frequent urination or even incontinence.

The Kidneys are also responsible for producing Marrow, but not the type of Marrow you read about in Western medical textbooks. In Eastern medicine, Marrow is a type of Blood that fills and nourishes your teeth, all of your bones, your spinal cord, and your brain. When your Kidneys are strong, you have healthy teeth and strong bones. Your mind is sharp and your thoughts are clear. When your Kidneys are weak, you are prone to tooth decay and brittle, porous bones. Your thinking dulls, your thoughts get foggy, and you start to notice that scourge of aging—forgetfulness.

Your Kidney Spirit

Just as the Kidneys oversee the span of time from birth to death, they also govern your mental and spiritual capacity to sustain the bigger picture of life—one's wisdom. This type of knowledge is greater than the brain's ability to store intellectual information. It is your deeper, spiritual connection into the unknown. Often infused in but not to be confused with one's religious faith or higher power, it is the realization that life exists on more than one level.

When your Kidneys are healthy, you are connected with and to your beliefs. Your mind can focus on goals and ambitions. If your Kidneys are weak, so is your mental willpower. Your mind can be easily swayed and your aspirations and dreams lost. When Kidney types lose their balance, their connection to their ethereal wisdom and intellectual knowledge weakens, like a brownout during a heat wave. It causes second guessing and self-doubt, which often creates a tremendous amount of fear.

This is what happened to Fran. Her loss of Kidney Qi balance created an irrational fear about her own health and the course her life was taking. The acupuncture I used to balance her Kidney Qi, along with her efforts to pay more attention to her diet, calmed her considerably. After several months of treatment, her hair stopped falling out, her skin and muscle tone returned, the darkness under her eyes lightened, her energy came back, her facial puffiness diminished, and once again she felt like her "old" youthful self.

CHARACTERISTICS OF A KIDNEY TYPE

Signs of healthy Kidneys are:

- A healthy, youthful appearance, no matter what age
- A thick, healthy head of hair
- A sturdy frame and dense physique
- Strong teeth and bones
- A sharp mind and clear thinking
- A strong spiritual connection

Signs of unhealthy Kidneys are:

- Premature aging
- A withered or puffy, pale appearance
- Dark circles under the eyes
- Early hair loss or premature graying
- Delayed growth and maturity
- Weak, brittle bones
- Dental problems
- Ringing in the ears or hearing loss
- Muddled thoughts and confusion
- Lack of ambition and goals
- Unexplainable or irrational fear

The Kidneys and the Evil Cold

The Kidneys are most affected by the evil known as cold. Cold injures your Kidneys. It can set in from overexposure to the cold outdoors, or something as seemingly harmless as sitting on a cold floor, or working in an open-air market in the wintertime. People who work in cold conditions, such as in an ice cream factory, butcher shop, or ice-skating rink, are prone to cold injury in their Kidneys.

The Kidneys are the "belly of your stove," so they need warmth. Your other Organs rely on their warmth in order to survive. Overexposure to cold conditions endangers not only the Kidneys but the health of the rest of your Organs as well. If the pilot light on a gas range goes out, the entire range goes cold. Your Kidneys are like the pilot light of your body. Without its constant warmth, the ability of your other Organs to maintain optimum health starts to diminish. The health of your Kidneys is so important, you can't survive without them.

Self-Acupressure for Building the Kidneys

We possess a finite amount of Kidney Qi. We are born with a specific amount of Kidney Qi to take us through life and acquire a limited supply of replenishable Qi from the foods we choose to eat and the lifestyle we choose to follow. Your goal, especially if you're a Kidney type, is to keep your Kidneys healthy and their Qi flowing.

Because Kidney health is so entwined in the aging process, the acupressure points involved in Kidney health are an integral part of the AcuFacial® Acupressure Facelift protocol that is the focal point of this book. However, there are many times in life when your Kidneys—and the way you look and feel—can benefit from concentrating on the self-acupressure routine given here.

Pay attention to your Kidneys when you're feeling mentally fatigued over an extended period of time, you have an illness you just can't shake, or you're under relentless stress—those times when your world gets rocked, as Fran's did.

The following routine concentrates on the lower limbs and face. Massage each point three times on both sides of the body in a clockwise rotation for ten seconds. Read the section "Touch and Go" starting on page 30 to learn the nuances of self-acupressure before beginning this massage.

ANKLES

Kidney 3 | K 3 is located in the soft spot on the inside of your ankle just above the foot, between the ankle bone and the tendon. This is the primary point for strengthening Kidney energy.

Kidney 6 | Move your finger toward the inside of your foot over and below the ankle bone. K 6 is the soft spot nearest the bone. This point is also used to strengthen Kidney energy.

Bladder 60 | BL 60 is located in the outside of your feet just below your ankle bone. This point is used to brighten the eyes and face. It also helps eliminate back pain.

Kidney 3

NECK

Bladder 10 | Place your fingers in the center of your spine, below the base of the skull. Slide your hands toward your ears until you land in a notch approximately one finger-width away. BL 10 opens the back of the neck to increase the flow of Qi and Blood to the head.

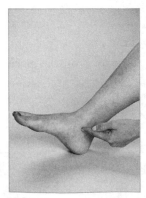

Kidney 6

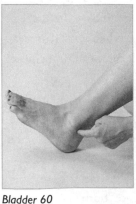

Bladder 60

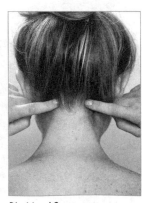

Bladder 10

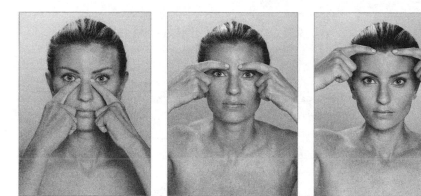

Bladder 1   Bladder 2   Bladder 3

FACE

Bladder 1 | BL 1 is located in the corner of your eye, on the side of the nose. It is used for all eye problems. It relaxes the eyes, soothes eyestrain, and alleviates eye puffiness and dark circles.

Bladder 2 | BL 2 is located at the inside ends of your eyebrows, above the inside corners of the eyes. It softens the forehead by releasing tension in the face and reducing creases between the eyebrows and forehead. It also helps relax the mind.

Bladder 3 | From BL 2, move your fingers straight up your forehead to the base of the hairline. This is BL 3. It relaxes forehead wrinkles.

The Anti-Aging Eating Strategy

As you go through this book, you'll notice that the dietary essentials for Kidney types contain a much larger selection of foods than for other Organs. There is a reason for this: Individual Organs generally prefer either Yin or Yang foods. Because the Kidneys supply the core energy to all the other Organs, the Kidneys depend on both Yin and Yang foods.

You can combine any Yang spice with any Yin food, or vice versa. For example, the Kidneys prefer that you add ginger (Yang) to fish (Yin), sesame oil (Yin) to string beans (Yang), or sprinkle cinnamon (Yang) on an apple

9-1-1 RESCUE THERAPY: HAIR LOSS

Poor Kidney Qi is really tough on your locks. The problem is exacerbated by stress and the use of hair dyes and harsh shampoos. The result is hair that loses its luster, thins, and starts to fall out.

In addition to the acupressure routine to restore Kidney Qi, you can help stop hair loss and strengthen your mane by reducing your stress through stress-reduction techniques, minimizing—or eliminating, if possible—the use of hair dyes, and using gentle hair products. In addition, you can use this ginger oil hair tonic. Ginger's potent stimulating properties help encourage circulation to the hair shafts and promote growth.

GINGER OIL HAIR TONIC

Ginger oil can be found in specialty stores, health food stores, and many supermarkets. If you can't find it, fresh ginger mixed into safflower oil will also work.

2 tablespoons ginger oil

or

2 tablespoons grated fresh ginger mixed into 2 tablespoons
    safflower oil

Rub the tonic into the scalp at the affected area or areas before bed every night for thirty days. Tie a scarf around your head or wear a shower cap to keep the oil from getting onto your bed linens.

(Yin). Combining Yin and Yang foods doesn't alter a food—it adds balance to your meal.

However, there are times when your diet needs to have more Yin or Yang. If you look puffy, often feel tired, and have chronic low back pain, you lack Yang and you should be eating Yang foods. If you are sallow and dry, get night sweats or flushing, or have brittle bones, you are lacking Yin and you should be eating Yin foods.

As you will see, most fish and fruit are Yin because, once consumed, they lubricate and moisten your face and Organs. Most spices are Yang because, after eating them, they remove puffiness from your face and tone your Organs.

ALWAYS REACH FOR SEA SALT

If you're a Kidney type, think salty. Salt is the taste that appeals to the Kidneys. On the surface, this appears to go against conventional wisdom because salt is considered a major dietary cause of water retention and puffiness, as well as certain health problems. However, there are two caveats to remember when you're reaching for the salt shaker: Think sea salt, and use it in moderation.

It's common knowledge that the human body is composed of about 75 percent water, but what is less known is that the water that keeps our cells nourished is salty like seawater.

This is why sea salt is vital to the Kidneys. It helps retain moisture in your body and kidneys, which in turn helps the bladder to move out impure fluids.

Sea salt is considered natural because it is nothing more than evaporated seawater. Regular table salt, on the other hand, is milled from underground salt deposits.

This is why all the recipes in this book call for sea salt. Consider sea salt good for the skin, especially if you're a Kidney type. However, like most other foods, it should be consumed in moderation.

The remaining categories are mixtures of Yin and Yang. Cooking food makes it more Yang, and eating it raw is more Yin. Keep in mind that, unless you specifically want to warm or cool your Kidneys, the key is *balance*, so when making your daily food choices, eat from both Yin and Yang.

Notice how your car doesn't run well in cold weather until the engine gets warm? Your body's engine, your Kidneys, also needs warmth to run smoothly, so it is best to eat foods that are heated or at room temperature. Keep cold and iced food and beverage consumption to a minimum, especially during winter, the Kidneys' vulnerable season. During the cold months, increase your consumption of sea salt and oil, which hydrates and protects your cells.

You should also avoid foods that are stimulants, such as coffee, chocolate, sugar, or anything else that produces an unnatural rush of energy. Stimulants

If you're a true Kidney type, you probably have a sophisticated palate, because many black foods are exotic. The Kidneys are nourished by foods that are colored black. Some are quite exotic but are readily available in upscale marketplaces, Asian or Indian markets, or in fine dining establishments. The health and nutrition benefits of black foods, especially the important role they play in Kidney health, are gaining popularity among chefs searching for unusual flavors for spectacular presentations. However, not all black foods lean toward the extraordinary. There are black foods to appeal to all tastes. Be on the lookout for these black foods:

- Black beans
- Blackberries
- Black currants
- Black grapes
- Black lentils
- Black olives
- Black raspberries
- Black rice
- Black sesame seeds
- Black tea (decaffeinated)
- Black trumpet mushrooms
- Black vinegar
- Blueberries
- Caviar
- Dates
- Figs
- Nori and other seaweed
- Shiitake mushrooms
- Soy sauce

have a negative effect on all Organs, but are especially stressful and taxing on the Kidneys.

Foods That Complement a Kidney Diet

Note: If you compare this list with other sources, you may find some discrepancies, as there is controversy as to whether some foods are considered Yin or Yang.

FISH, FOWL, MEAT

Pork is a Yin food that deserves a special place in a Kidney diet because it directly nourishes your Kidneys. This is why you'll find two pork recipes in this chapter.

These foods are Yin:

- Abalone
- Bluefish
- Catfish
- Caviar
- Chicken eggs
- Clams
- Crab
- Cuttlefish
- Duck
- Kidney (organic)
- Mussels
- Oysters
- Pork
- Pork sausage
- Rabbit
- Shrimp
- Trout
- Tuna

These foods are Yang:

- Beef
- Lamb
- Lobster
- Mutton
- Octopus
- Venison

VEGETABLES

These vegetables are Yin:

- Artichokes
- Asparagus
- Beets
- Beet greens
- Cabbage (red)
- Cucumbers
- Fava beans
- Peas
- Pickled vegetables
- Pickles
- Radicchio
- Sea vegetables (particularly arame, hijiki, kelp, kombu, nori, and wakame)
- Sweet potatoes
- Tomatoes
- Yams

These vegetables are Yang:

- Fennel
- Onions
- Potatoes (white)
- Shiitake mushrooms
- Squash (all types)
- String beans

FRUIT

The majority of fruits are Yin:

- Apples
- Apricots
- Avocados
- Bananas
- Bayberries
- Blackberries
- Boysenberries
- Coconut milk
- Cranberries
- Dates
- Figs
- Grapes (black)
- Lemons
- Loquats
- Mandarin oranges
- Mangos
- Oranges
- Pears
- Pineapples
- Plums
- Pomegranates
- Strawberries
- Tomatoes
- Watermelons

These fruits are Yang:

- Cherries
- Coconut meat
- Peaches
- Raspberries

GRAINS

These grains are Yin:

- Barley
- Buckwheat

These grains are Yang:

- Millet
- Rice (black, glutinous, white, and wild)
- Whole wheat flour

LEGUMES

These legumes are Yin:

- Adzuki beans
- Kidney beans
- Mung beans
- Tofu

These legumes are Yang:
- Black beans
- Peanuts

This legume is neutral (both Yin and Yang):
- Black soybeans

NUTS AND SEEDS

These nuts and seeds are Yin:
- Black sesame seeds
- Lychee nuts
- Pine nuts
- Water chestnuts

These nuts and seeds are Yang:
- Chestnuts
- Dill seeds
- Pistachios
- Walnuts

OILS

Oil is lubricating, so you want to make sure to get it in your diet. All oils are Yin, except for olive oil, which is both Yin and Yang. Stick with healthy oils; favor these:

- Canola oil
- Olive oil (all varieties)
- Sesame oil

BEVERAGES

Stay away from beverages that are cold and contain caffeine. You can make warming teas by steeping spices from the Yang condiments and spices category.

- Clove tea
- Spearmint tea

CONDIMENTS AND SPICES

These condiments and spices are Yin:

- Agave nectar
- Black vinegar
- Honey
- Miso
- Parsley

- Peppermint
- Royal jelly
- Sea salt
- Sugar (white)
- Worcestershire sauce

These condiments and spices are Yang:

- Anise
- Bay leaves
- Black pepper
- Cayenne pepper
- Chives
- Cinnamon
- Cloves
- Curry powder
- Fennel seeds
- Fenugreek seeds

- Garlic
- Ginger
- Horseradish
- Nutmeg
- Rosemary
- Sage
- Spearmint
- Star anise
- Thyme
- Turmeric

The Three-Day Kidney Menu

Balancing the diet with foods that are Yin and Yang takes a little practice, but once you get familiar with the foods in each category, developing your menus is easy. This three-day sample menu offers a combination of Yin and Yang foods for Kidney health. Feel free to Yang them up or Yin them down.

DAY 1

BREAKFAST

Fruit cup

Omelet with mushrooms and chives

Clove or peppermint tea

LUNCH

> *Pork Tenderloin (page 73)*
> *Lemon Asparagus (page 73)*
> Sliced tomato with extra virgin olive oil and rosemary

DINNER

> Tossed green salad with extra virgin olive oil and black vinegar
> *Linguine with Lobster and Garlic (page 75)*
> Steamed green beans with black sesame seeds
> Fresh or dried dates

DAY 2

BREAKFAST

> Grape and mandarin orange cup
> Eggs, any style
> Whole wheat toast
> Decaffeinated hot tea or coffee

LUNCH

> Shrimp, any style
> String beans
> Steamed brown rice
> Watermelon

DINNER

> *Pork Sausage with Black Beans (page 72)*
> *Baked Acorn Squash (page 74)*
> *Dark Fruit Salad (page 75)*

DAY 3

BREAKFAST

> Sliced avocado and tomato on whole wheat toast
> Tropical fruit cup
> Cinnamon tea

LUNCH

> *Vegetable Barley Soup (page 77)*
> Whole grain roll

DINNER

Roast Leg of Lamb with Garlic and Rosemary (page 76) with horseradish
sauce

Steamed artichoke

Wild rice

Sliced pineapple

Rejuvenating Recipes

*Each of these recipes contains a balance of Yin and Yang foods especially tailored
for Kidney health.*

PORK SAUSAGE WITH BLACK BEANS

*Kidney types who like sausage should favor pork sausage because pork is so good for
the Kidneys.*

8 pork sausage links
1 16-ounce can black beans, with liquid
1 small onion, chopped
1 garlic clove, minced
¼ teaspoon cayenne pepper
2 tablespoons chopped fresh cilantro
Sea salt, to taste

1 Put the sausages in a skillet large enough to hold them in one layer and cover
   with water. Bring to a simmer over medium heat, cover, and cook until most of
   the water has evaporated, about 10 minutes. Set aside to cool.

2 Combine the black beans with their liquid, the onion, garlic, and cayenne in a
   medium saucepan and bring to a boil. Reduce the heat, add the sausage links,
   and simmer until heated through, about 5 minutes. Divide the sausage links
   among 4 plates and spoon the beans on the side. Sprinkle with the cilantro.
   Season with salt if desired.

SERVES 4

▨ PORK TENDERLOIN

I 2- to 3-pound pork tenderloin
I tablespoon olive oil
I teaspoon dried rosemary
I teaspoon garlic powder
½ teaspoon sea salt
½ teaspoon cayenne pepper

1 Rinse the tenderloin in cold water and pat dry. Rub all sides with ½ tablespoon of the oil.

2 Combine the rosemary, garlic powder, salt, and cayenne and rub all over the tenderloin.

3 Heat the remaining ½ tablespoon oil in a heavy-bottomed Dutch oven over high heat for 2 minutes, making sure it covers the bottom and sides. Put the tenderloin in the skillet and brown it for about I minute on each side, rotating the meat until it is browned all over.

4 Lower the heat to medium-low, cover, and cook, rotating frequently, 15 to 20 minutes, until the pork reaches a temperature of 155°F. Remove from the heat, cover loosely with foil, and let sit for 10 minutes before slicing.

SERVES 4

▨ LEMON ASPARAGUS

For this simple side dish, use the thinnest asparagus you can find. Asparagus is all Yin. Serve hot or cold.

I bunch thin-stemmed asparagus
I lemon
Dash of sea salt

Remove the bottom stalks of the asparagus spears at the point where they snap. Steam until tender. Remove to a bowl, squeeze the lemon over the asparagus, and season with the salt.

SERVES 4

⊞ FRESH FENNEL SALAD

This recipe illustrates how easy it is to balance Yin (lemon and parsley) with Yang (fennel), and the oil is neutral. Fennel has a strong anise-like flavor and can be eaten cooked or raw.

> 1 fennel bulb
> 2 tablespoons extra virgin olive oil
> 1 tablespoon fresh lemon juice
> 1 tablespoon chopped fresh flat-leaf parsley
> Sea salt and freshly ground black pepper to taste

1 Remove the leafy stalk from the fennel bulb and slice the bulb very thin with a mandoline or in a food processor. Transfer the fennel to a salad bowl.

2 Whisk together the remaining ingredients in a medium bowl. Add the dressing to the fennel and mix to coat.

SERVES 4

⊞ BAKED ACORN SQUASH

Agave nectar is a natural sweetener that is low on the glycemic index, meaning it won't contribute to a spike in insulin. It is available is most supermarkets; if you can't find it, substitute honey.

> 1 medium acorn squash
> 1 tablespoon unsalted butter
> 1 tablespoon agave nectar
> Pinch of ground cinnamon
> Sea salt and freshly ground black pepper

1 Preheat the oven to 375°F.

2 Cut the squash in half and remove the seeds.

3 Place the squash halves on a cookie sheet, flesh side down, and bake for 45 minutes.

4 Transfer the squash halves, flesh side up, into a deep baking dish large enough to hold them snuggly. Place half of the butter and agave in the center of each half. Sprinkle with the cinnamon and season with the salt and pepper. Cover and bake for another 45 minutes, until tender when pierced with a fork. Slice each half in two pieces and serve.

SERVES 4

▨ DARK FRUIT SALAD

Meyer lemons are sweeter and less acidic than regular lemons, and they have a slight orange flavor. If you can't find them, substitute regular lemons. The salad won't taste the same, but it will still be delicious.

> 8 fresh dates, pitted and cut in half
> 1 cup fresh blueberries
> 1 cup seedless black grapes, cut in half
> 3 black plums, pitted and quartered
> 8 fresh figs, quartered
> ½ Meyer lemon

Combine the first five ingredients in a glass bowl. Squeeze the lemon juice over the fruit and stir to coat. Let the fruit sit at room temperature for 30 minutes before serving.

SERVES 4

▨ LINGUINE WITH LOBSTER AND GARLIC

Lobster is one of the few types of seafood with a Yang property. When combined with the Yin foods in this recipe, it creates a perfect tasty balance.

> ½ pound whole wheat linguine
> ½ cup extra virgin olive oil
> 6 cloves garlic, finely chopped

½ cup fresh flat-leaf parsley
1½ cups canned diced tomatoes, with juice
½ cup dry white wine
1 pound lobster meat, cooked
½ teaspoon sea salt
Freshly ground black pepper

1 Bring a large pot of salted water to a boil, add the pasta, and cook according to the package directions until it is al dente, about 8 minutes. Drain and set aside.

2 Heat the oil in a large skillet over high heat. Reduce the heat to medium-low and add the garlic and ¼ cup of the parsley. Sauté gently until the garlic is soft but not browned, about 1 minute.

3 Add the diced tomatoes with their juice to the pan and simmer, uncovered, until the tomatoes start to form a thick sauce, about 10 minutes. Pour in the wine and continue to cook for 3 minutes.

4 Add the lobster, stir, cover the pan, and cook until warmed through, about 30 seconds. Add the linguine, salt, and pepper to taste and stir for about 1 minute, until heated through. Garnish with the remaining ¼ cup parsley.

SERVES 4

ROAST LEG OF LAMB WITH GARLIC AND ROSEMARY

Serve this roast with horseradish sauce or a traditional mint sauce.

1 boneless lamb roast (about 6 pounds)
3 or 4 garlic cloves, peeled and slivered
1 tablespoon ketchup
1 tablespoon Worcestershire sauce
Juice of 1 large lemon
1 tablespoon chopped fresh rosemary
2 teaspoons sea salt
2 teaspoons freshly ground black pepper
1 large carrot, peeled and cut into 4 pieces

1 medium onion, quartered
1 celery stalk, cut into four pieces
1 to 2 tablespoons extra virgin olive oil

1 Wash and pat dry the lamb and tie with roasting string. With a sharp paring knife, make several slits about ½ inch into the flesh of the lamb all around. Push a sliver of garlic into each of the slits. Place the roast in a baking pan.

2 To make the marinade, combine the ketchup, Worcestershire sauce, lemon juice, rosemary, salt, and pepper in a small bowl. Rub the marinade all over the roast. Let the roast sit at room temperature for 1 hour or cover and refrigerate overnight.

3 Preheat the oven to 425°F.

4 Put the carrot, onion, and celery in a small bowl. Add the oil and stir to coat the vegetables evenly. Scatter the vegetables around the roast.

5 Put the roast in the oven and roast for 20 minutes. Lower the temperature to 325°F and continue to roast for 1 hour, or until it reaches your desired doneness. Let rest before slicing and serving.

SERVES 6 TO 8

VEGETABLE BARLEY SOUP

With this soup, it couldn't be easier to warm the Kidneys on a cold winter day.

2 quarts vegetable broth
1 cup uncooked pearl barley
2 large carrots, peeled and chopped
2 celery stalks, chopped
1 14.5-ounce can diced tomatoes, with juice
1 zucchini, chopped
1 15-ounce can adzuki beans, drained
1 onion, chopped
1 teaspoon Worcestershire sauce
1 teaspoon garlic powder
1 teaspoon sugar
1 teaspoon sea salt

½ teaspoon ground black pepper

1 teaspoon dried parsley

1 teaspoon curry powder

1 teaspoon paprika

3 bay leaves

Pour the vegetable broth into a large pot. Add the remaining ingredients and bring to a boil. Reduce the heat, cover, and simmer for about 90 minutes, until the soup is very thick. If it is too thick, thin it out by adding more broth. Remove the bay leaves before serving.

SERVES 8

Natural Anti-Aging Formulas

I challenge anyone to say that at the very least they have not been tempted to try one of the myriad anti-aging creams and lotions advertised just about everywhere. Anti-aging creams and formulas are *big* business. This is why, in order to stay young, we fill our bathroom cabinets with antioxidant concoctions and our refrigerators with brews that fight free radicals.

But what claims can you believe and which ones should you take with a grain of salt? That's a difficult question to answer, but I can say that keeping your skin youthful means you must keep it nourished. This means you should be looking for a serum.

Anti-aging serums are concentrated sources of active ingredients that work into the deeper layers of your skin. All skin care products are made up of active ingredients and inactive ingredients. Active ingredients are those that work directly on your skin. Vitamins A and E and antioxidants with known anti-aging and skin-protecting action are among the most common active ingredients found in good anti-aging serums. Algae is another well-researched active ingredient; it is used to revitalize and replenish the skin with minerals. Plant products, such as certain herbs, fruits, and saps from specific varieties of trees, contain phytohormones, which have proven skin-healing and skin-soothing properties.

Inactive ingredients don't target the skin; they are included in serum formulations to give consistency and add to shelf life. Examples of inactive ingredients are preservatives (methylparaben), colorants (dyes or pigments), fragrance (perfumes), substances that hold the product together (glycerin), and base substances (alcohol and water).

Although many products use artificial or chemically derived active and inactive ingredients, there are now many effective "green" or organically certified and eco-certified products on the market today, and I am glad to see it. This means that these products contain no artificial ingredients or harmful preservatives. In the case of eco-certification, the environments in which the products are produced and packaged also adhere to stringent green regulations.

Of all skin care products, serums have the highest amount of active ingredients, which is why they are also the most expensive. They can range in price up to hundreds of dollars or more. And you can't expect to get much for your money, because the active ingredients in anti-aging serums are concentrated, tend to have a short shelf life, and are therefore sold in small quantities. However, a little goes a long way; most serums are formulated so it takes only a few drops to get all-over coverage.

Make-It-Yourself Serums with Essential Oils

You can save quite a bit of money by making your own formulas using essential oils, highly concentrated droplets from the flowers, leaves, stems, roots, or bark of botanical plants. When you brush against a lavender plant or put a geranium to your nose, you are taking in the plant's essence, unique as a fingerprint. Some of the best serums on the market contain essential oils.

Essential oils are extremely potent. Some oils can be one hundred times more potent than the plants from which they are extracted. They also have been scientifically proven to contain strong healing characteristics, with many containing anti-aging properties. So you can see why essentials oils can make excellent serums.

Essentials oils are also quite volatile, meaning they will turn from liquid to gas readily when exposed to light and air. To protect the homemade serums featured here, store them in a clean, amber-colored bottle with a tight-fitting lid and keep them in a cool place out of direct sunlight, since they contain no preservatives and can become rancid if kept too long. Essential oils can be found in health food stores, most pharmacies, and at the beauty counters of many department stores.

Essential oils must be mixed with a carrier oil in order to make a serum.

Following are a few make-it-yourself serums that I have found work well. Make your serums weekly and shake them well before using.

To use these oils, put two or three drops in the palm of your hand and massage into your face and neck every morning after washing your face and before applying makeup. Use again at bedtime as the final step in your skin care routine. Increase or decrease the ingredient proportions to suit your desired consistency or result. Before using any product, whether homemade or purchased, I recommend performing a skin allergy patch test (page 219).

GARDEN OF EDEN

This anti-aging formula is designed to energize dry to normal skin. The almond and evening primrose oils are rich in essential fatty acids that hydrate dry skin. Calendula and palmarosa essential oils are soothing and nourishing, and geranium oil brings a radiant glow to your skin.

I tablespoon almond oil
I tablespoon evening primrose oil
10 drops calendula essential oil
10 drops palmarosa essential oil
5 drops geranium essential oil
3 drops lavender essential oil

Place the almond and evening primrose oils in a dark or amber glass jar. Add the essential oils.

Shake gently and apply to the skin as directed above and as needed.

FRUITS OF HEAVEN

This is a wonderful serum for older, wrinkled skin and is good for all skin types. Apricot kernel oil is a rich oil high in essential fatty acids. Carrot seed removes excess water retention and nourishes the skin. Neroli oil relaxes the skin, while lemon and orange oils reduce skin wrinkling. Geranium oil adds radiance to your complexion.

2 tablespoons apricot kernel oil
10 drops carrot seed essential oil

10 drops blue chamomile essential oil
8 drops neroli essential oil
5 drops geranium essential oil
5 drops lemon essential oil
4 drops orange essential oil

Place the apricot kernel oil in a dark or amber glass jar. Add the essential oils. Shake gently and apply to the skin as directed above and as needed.

◫ EYE SEE YOU

This is a great eye oil for puffiness and dark shadows under the eyes. When using this formula, it is important that you test for an allergic reaction first on a small area on the skin, such as your wrist or the inside of your elbow. Since the skin around the eye is delicate, use with caution until you know you can use it safely.

1 teaspoon hazelnut oil
8 drops carrot essential oil
8 drops German chamomile essential oil
8 drops rose essential oil

Place the hazelnut oil in a dark or amber glass jar. Add the essential oils. Shake gently and apply to skin as directed above and as needed.

IF YOU DON'T WANT TO MAKE IT, THEN BUY IT . . .

The following products are my favorite serums. Use them after cleansing and toning. I have used them all, and love them.

Yon-Ka Paris Serum
Cost: About $53
Size: .5 oz.
This vitamin-rich face oil repairs, nourishes, and boosts aging skin. It combats free radicals that are responsible for the aging process. Apply 2 to 3 pumps morning and night, alone or added to your daytime moisturizer or night preparation product. Make sure you use enough serum to saturate the skin properly.

Kiehl's Açaí Damage-Repairing Serum

Cost: About $49

Size: 1.7 oz.

This is a lightweight formula that quickly penetrates into your skin. With repeated use it helps repair the effects of visible damage to skin tone, texture, and elasticity.

Naturopathica Plant Stem Cell Serum

Cost: About $48

Size: .5 oz.

Swiss scientists discovered that ingredients derived from the wound-healing tissue of plants (stem cells) can improve human cell health and vitality. Stem cells from echinacea, butterfly bush, açaí, and helichrysum plants are used to slow cell aging as a result of harmful sun rays and cell damage. You can actually feel it tightening your skin.

Radical Skincare Youth Infusion Serum

Cost: About $140

Size: 30 ml

This anti-aging serum contains the perfect blend of ingredients for lifting and moisturizing. It uses antioxidants from açaí berry, grapeseed extract, green tea, and coffeeberry and resveratrol (found in grapes and wine) to firm aging skin, reduce fine lines and wrinkles, enhance skin luminosity, and visibly tighten sagging skin. Hyaluronic acid, a lubricant that is naturally made in your body, is added to hydrate dry skin.

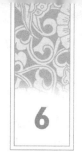

6

Bags and Sags: Portrait of a Spleen Face

AT AGE FORTY-ONE, REESE SAID SHE FELT THE way she looked—"droopy and tired." She had creases from her nose to mouth that were deep for her age. She was considering cosmetic fillers but kept putting it off because she was uncomfortable about having foreign substances injected into her body. She read about my cosmetic procedure in a beauty magazine and decided the natural route was her way to go.

Round and full-figured, Reese looked puffy in the face and said she often felt bloated. As we talked, I found out that Reese suffered from indigestion, especially after meals. She was also unhappy about her weight. Although she craved sugar and starches, she watched what she ate and tried to stick to a low-fat diet. She complained that she has always had trouble losing weight. She explained that on a "good day," her diet consisted of fruit and yogurt for breakfast; salad with chicken or another protein for lunch; and protein, steamed vegetables, and more salad for dinner. But it didn't seem to matter what she ate. She wasn't losing weight. To make matters worse, she said she

SNAPSHOT OF THE
SPLEEN

Element: Earth

Complementary Organ: Stomach

Primary function: Maintaining muscle tone

Facial concern: Sagging muscles

Emotional regulation: Worry

Complementary orifice: Mouth

Season: Changing of season

Color: Yellow

Taste: Sweet

Primary evil: Dampness

Active time: 7 a.m. to 11 a.m.

just "didn't feel right." She felt like she was mentally in a fog and had difficulty making decisions. She confided that much of her fatigue, both physical and mental, could probably be blamed on her tendency as an enabler. She just had trouble saying no to others who wanted a share of her time.

It didn't take much investigating to figure out that Reese had the classic signs of Spleen Qi deficiency.

Profile of a Spleen Type

Healthy Spleen types have strong, thick face muscles, a smooth, glowing complexion, a round physique, and a natural affinity to firm body tone. They are down-to-earth, friendly, and nurturing. Spleen types are peacemakers. They embody sympathy and caring and will readily advocate for those in need, whatever the cause may be. They crave a harmonious environment and wish peace and goodwill to all. Healthy Spleen types are loyal, giving, and reliable.

When Spleen types get out of balance, however, you can see it in their looks and actions. Like the Pillsbury Dough Boy, they tend to get soft and puffy. They get swelling around their eyes, their cheek and jowl muscles sag, and the skin on their neck starts to hang. Their body shape becomes round and full figured—the apple shape you often read and hear about. Their normally soft and smooth skin breaks out, especially around the mouth and chin. They bruise easily.

Lethargy is part of the package of an out-of-whack Spleen. So, too, are digestive problems. Bloating is common, and Spleen types frequently complain about heaviness in their abdomen, arms, and legs. They are prone to sinus problems and frequently have allergies. Difficulty losing weight is a classic symptom of an unhealthy Spleen. Female Spleen types are also prone to cellulite.

When Spleen types get out of balance, they become worriers, and can be meddling, overprotective, obsessive, and self-doubting.

The Role of the Spleen: Healthy Muscles

Out of all the Organs, when your Spleen gets out of balance, it shows up most in the health of your muscles in both your face and your body. This is because the Spleen is responsible for nourishing the muscles of your face, arms, and legs, and for maintaining good overall muscle tone. Although exercise will improve the fitness and contour of your muscles, it affects only the muscles you actively work, and your face muscles are not usually on a trainer's agenda! However, when you have a strong Spleen, your face muscles are naturally firm, contoured, and lifted. The muscles of your arms are naturally well shaped and your leg muscles are sculpted and strong. In fact, a healthy Spleen type might even have an advantage over other Organ types when it comes to body sculpting through physical activities, such as yoga, dance-type exercise routines, and resistance training.

When your Spleen becomes weak, facial muscles start to lose their natural tone. They become heavy and puffy and start to sag. You may notice jowls that didn't exist before, formed by a deepening crease from the nose to the mouth (what is technically called the nasolabial fold), and the mouth to the chin—the primary reason Reese showed up in my office.

The muscles in your arms and legs also start to lose their firmness. Initially, they may feel heavy and tired. Over time they become flabby. Then they begin to wiggle and jiggle. Upper arms start to sag, creating the unflattering sight of what many refer to as batwings. Suddenly women want to

---

FUNCTIONS OF THE SPLEEN

The Spleen teams up with the Stomach to perform these key functions:

- Transform food and beverages into energy for the body
- Oversee the health and tone quality of muscles
- Control the need to worry constantly
- Keep Blood in the vessels
- Influence how we think and our ability to think
- Keep lips moist and rosy

cover up their arms, even at the beach, and shun the sleeveless and strapless clothes in their closets.

A damaged Spleen is also the primary cause of cellulite, strands of muscle and fat under the skin of the thighs and elsewhere that have the unsightly external appearance of lumpy cottage cheese.

The Causes of a Spleen Imbalance

The Spleen's ability to function properly can be affected in many ways, including by other Organs. If the Stomach isn't working properly, if Kidney Qi is weak, if the Lungs can't grab Qi essence, if the Heart can't absorb Blood essence, or if the Liver is overactive, the Spleen is affected. Weak Spleen is also caused by a poor diet, a diet high in foods that aggravate your Organ type, or other unhealthy eating habits.

People who live near the ocean or in areas of near-constant humidity, such as the Deep South, or who work in a damp, cool environment, such as plumbers and miners, or even people who work in a basement office, are prone to Spleen problems.

Are you a worrywart? If so, it usually is not hard to tell, because worriers wear their emotions on their face. Western doctors will tell you that excessive worry is a cause for the kind of unhealthy stress that can weaken the heart, but Eastern doctors explain it by blaming it on the harmful effect it has on your Spleen. Yes, excessive worrying can damage the Spleen.

Westerners believe that over time the muscles of your face change shape,

---

HOW A FACE "UNFOLDS"

Photos in chapter 1 (pages 10 and 11) illustrate how weak cheek muscles can change your appearance. When cheek muscles lose their tone, they begin to sag. This creates the nasolabial fold, which extends from the nose to the mouth, and makes you look tired. When muscles between the eyes and across the forehead get tight, it creates what is called the glabellar crease, which makes you look angry.

that it is a natural part of the aging process. Easterners believe it is caused by an unhealthy Spleen.

As time passes, continual use of the same expressions (think of the frown of a constant worrier and the lip lines of someone who smokes), normal gravitational pull, and years of poor posture (a common characteristic of many people, especially those carrying excess weight) cause the head to shift forward and the chin to drop downward, causing the large band of muscles of your neck to contract and shorten. The muscles of your neck are attached at one end to your collarbone and on the other end to the muscles surrounding the lower portion of your face and mouth. Over time, tight neck muscles pull on the muscles of your lower face and mouth, which then pull and stretch your cheek and eye muscles. In addition, the band of muscles across your forehead and the smaller muscles between your eyebrows become tense and tight.

The Link to Healthy Digestion

The hallmark of a strong Spleen is healthy digestion. Our well-being depends upon the body's ability to absorb and process nourishment, and this is the role of the Spleen. The Spleen takes the foods and liquids we ingest and extracts their vital nutrients to begin the important process of transforming them into Qi and Blood and transporting them to other Organs. The Spleen then sends what the body can't use downward to the Stomach, where it is digested and then eliminated.

When the Spleen is weak, its ability to transform and transport nutrients becomes impaired, and it can't do its job. Good goes down, bad goes up. The result is poor digestion, gas, and bloating. Not only can you feel it, but you can see it as sagging facial muscles.

In addition, the Spleen keeps Blood in the vessels or pathways that travel throughout your body. When your Spleen is weak, its ability to keep the Blood in their vessels is compromised. As a result, the Blood can seep from the vessels to the surface of the skin, which means you can bruise easily. Because the Spleen rules the mouth, a weak Spleen means your lips get pale and dry and you can develop a yellowish cast around your mouth.

The Spleen and Its Evil: Dampness

In order to do its primary job of sorting food properly, the Spleen needs to be dry. When the Spleen gets weak, it is prone to the Eastern medicine evil known as dampness.

Although anyone can have a damp Spleen, it is most problematic in people exposed to a moist environment, such as those who live in geographic locations where there is a lot of moisture in the air, and in people who work in humid or moist conditions.

When the walls of your house get wet and don't have an opportunity to

---

9-1-1 RESCUE THERAPY: ALLERGIES, CELLULITE, AND A WEIGHT PROBLEM

When Spleen dampness sets in and isn't corrected, the moisture in your body begins to thicken like gelatin. As dampness begins to accumulate, it manifests as other physical problems.

Allergies: Is your nose always stuffed up? Congestion is a classic symptom of a damp Spleen, and you can feel it in your sinuses. A seriously compromised Spleen can cry out as a chronic seasonal or food allergy, or even as asthma. Correct your Spleen and see your allergies diminish. They may even disappear.

Cellulite: Cellulite is *not* an inevitable part of aging. But it is an inevitable result of a Spleen damaged by too much dampness. It forms its unflattering dimpling pattern on the arms, legs, hips, butt, stomach, and midriff. Correct the Spleen and see your cellulite fade away.

Weight gain: Wonder why some people can eat and eat and not gain weight, yet you feel you can gain weight just by looking at food? Blame it on your Spleen. The Spleen's job is to begin the process of changing food and drink into nourishment. When it can't do its job properly, you become sluggish and can't lose weight. An unhealthy Spleen also loses its ability to send what it doesn't need to the Stomach to break down and eliminate, which is why some people are plagued by chronic indigestion, bloating, and gas, which can further impede the ability to lose weight. A struggle with weight is a problem caused by Spleen dampness. Correct your Spleen, adjust your diet, and watch those extra pounds disappear.

---

dry, eventually they develop a type of mold called mildew. If left untreated, mildew spreads and eventually damages your walls. The same is true with your body. Frequent exposure to damp conditions causes your Spleen to become damp, making you look and feel puffy. As dampness accumulates in the Spleen, it damages the Organ's ability to function properly.

It is no stretch of the imagination to understand that the dampness and moisture surrounding the body can settle within. From the perspective of your Spleen, this is not a good thing. Just thinking about it can give you a chill.

Seeing Life with Clarity

The Spleen governs mental clarity. Similar to the way the Spleen processes food, it digests thoughts as well. Your ability to focus, concentrate, and think is connected to this Organ. The Spleen governs nourishment and feelings of concern for self and others.

When the Spleen is strong, you are able to nourish yourself emotionally and also give appropriate nourishment to others. When you eat well, sleep comfortably, stay fit, and live with integrity, your thoughts are clear and focused, and you can make clear decisions—all because your Spleen is strong and healthy.

When the Spleen is unhealthy, however, these attributes begin to skew. Rather than being nurturing, you may come across as bossy or controlling. You can even obsess about your need to help others. A good example is motherhood taken too far. We've all seen it, if not experienced it. It is natural for a mother to dote over her infant and toddler—feeding, clothing, protecting, and, yes, even fretting. As a child grows into a teen and young adult, a mother's love and concern for health and safety can be just as strong, but there is a time to let go, when it is no longer appropriate or healthy for her to continually make her children's meals, wash their clothes, supervise their wardrobes, wait up for them at night, and constantly tell them what to do.

The inability to separate and adhere to these kinds of appropriate boundaries is indicative of a weak Spleen.

Life itself is a reflection of a healthy Spleen, and the Spleen is the mirror of your self-worth. Everything that we see, smell, and hear gets assimilated through the Spleen. If your Spleen is well nourished, you have a deep inner

CHARACTERISTICS OF A SPLEEN TYPE

Signs of a healthy Spleen are:

- Firm, sculpted cheeks and jawline
- Even skin coloring
- Toned arms and legs

- Healthy digestion
- Friendly, reliable, nurturing, peacekeeping attributes
- Self-assuredness

Signs of an unhealthy Spleen are:

- Muscle sagging in the cheeks and jawline
- Heaviness in the limbs
- Brownish-yellow spots on the skin
- Easy bruising
- Sallow, yellowish skin tone, particularly around the mouth
- Pale, dry, or cracked lips
- Sinus congestion
- Digestion problems
- Inability to lose or gain weight

- Cellulite
- Weak muscle tone
- Excessive worrying
- Obsessive thinking
- Confusion
- Indecisiveness
- Always putting others before self
- Constantly seeking the approval of others
- Lack of good self-esteem

feeling of well-being and a strong sense of security. On the other hand, if your Spleen is weak, you may find yourself constantly seeking the approval of others for self-validation.

Mental clarity and self-esteem are reflected in your facial expression and body language. When your mind is clear and you feel good about yourself, your face is open and lifted and your posture is erect. If you are feeling confused and unsure of yourself, your head and face muscles droop and your body slumps forward.

Self-Acupressure for Saggy Cheeks

This acupressure routine is the same acupuncture routine I used on Reese and that I use on other Spleen types with a deficiency. It will help you restore your Spleen Qi and noticeably lift and tone your cheek muscles, brighten your complexion, and make you feel more energized. If you are troubled by sagging cheeks, you can spend extra time on these points in the Acu-Facial® Acupressure Facelift protocol, or use it as a stand-alone treatment. You should see and feel noticeable results within twenty days. In this massage, you start with the legs, then work your way to the hands, neck, and face. Read the section "Touch and Go: Key Acupressure Points (page 30) before beginning this routine.

LEGS

Work the points on each leg using your index finger and applying medium pressure by rotating your finger clockwise in a circular motion for approximately ten rotations. You can work the legs individually or both at the same time, though this can be a little tricky, as it is important for the motion to be clockwise. Do the complete leg sequence, then repeat two more times.

Spleen 3 | SP 3 is located on the inside of your foot, below the head of the large toe, on the edge of the dark and light skin. This is the primary point for strengthening weak Spleen Qi and eliminating Spleen dampness. Massage it to address sagging muscles.

Spleen 6 | SP 6 is located on the inside of the leg, roughly four finger-widths above the top of the ankle bone. It is the intersection of all Yin leg

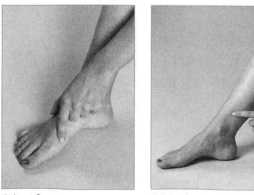

Spleen 3   Spleen 6

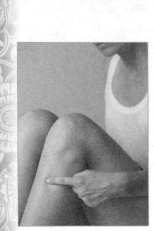

Stomach 36

Meridians. In addition to lifting facial and body muscles, it balances and strengthens the Qi and Blood of the Spleen, Liver, and Kidney.

Stomach 36 | Next move to pressure point ST 36, located in the depression four finger-widths below the bottom of the outside of the knee bone. In addition to lifting the cheek muscles, this point also strengthens the digestive system, supports the immune system, and improves physical stamina.

Spleen 10 | To locate SP 10, place the palm of your hand on the bottom of the opposite knee with the thumb extended upward. Your thumb should fall into a depression above the knee on the inside of the leg. This point stimulates blood flow.

HEAD AND FACE POINTS

Follow the same instructions as for the legs and arms, though you should lighten up on the pressure a bit when you get to the face. Massage these points in sequence, then repeat two more times.

Triple Heater 17 | Move your fingers to the depression behind the ear below the skull. This is point TH 17. This point drains congestion from the head. It clears lymphatic congestion and is particularly good for sinus congestion, facial swelling, and skin problems. It is also used to loosen the muscles of the neck.

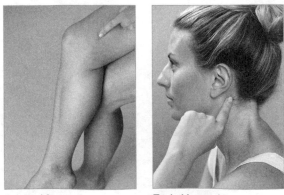

Spleen 10　　　　*Triple Heater 17*

Stomach 3 through Stomach 7 | Don't let the word *stomach* mislead you. All these points are located on the face and, when combined in this specific pattern, are the primary points for lifting cheek muscles. Since the points are not arranged in order, it is important to pay attention to the instructions.

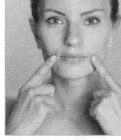

Stomach 4 | ST 4 is located below the center of your eye at the level of the corner of your mouth.

Stomach 5 | ST 5 is located above the jawline, one finger-width in front of ST 6. With ST 4 and ST 6 it relaxes the jaw and tightens the jawline.

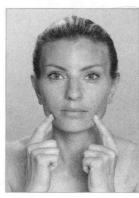
Stomach 4

Stomach 6 | ST 6 is located one finger-width above and behind the angle of the jaw.

Stomach 7 | Now move your fingers in front of your ear. You can find ST 7 by feeling for the depression at the intersection of the lower border of the cheekbone and the upper corner of the jawbone.

Stomach 3 | ST 3 is located directly below the center of your eye at the level of the nostrils.

Stomach 5

Small Intestine 18 | SI 18 is located on the cheek, directly below the outer edge of the eye and to the side of the nose. It is added to this sequence to lift and sculpt the cheekbone.

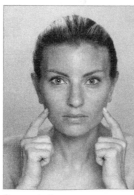
Stomach 6

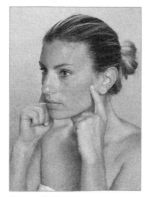
Stomach 7

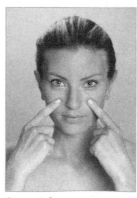
Stomach 3

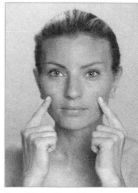
Small Intestine 18

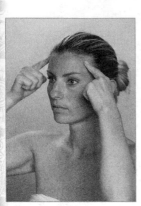

Stomach 8

Stomach 8 | ST 8 is located at the edge of the forehead at the bend in your hairline. It lifts the muscles of the cheek and forehead.

Eating to Lift Saggy Cheeks and Improve Muscle Tone

Chewing is the signal that kicks the Spleen into action to transform what you are eating into usable Qi. Your food choices and how well you chew your food influence how effectively the Spleen does its job.

Because the Spleen is so involved with digestion, your dietary habits influence its health more than any other Organ. This means that Spleen types are more vulnerable to the effects of food and suffer more from overindulgence and other dietary abuses.

An unhealthy Spleen diet can cause Spleen dampness. Overindulging in damp-producing foods affects the Spleen, and a steady diet of these foods over time can cause the chronic complaints associated with Spleen weakness, including saggy facial muscles and the other cosmetic problems already described. Eating too many cold, raw, or fried foods—even healthy foods such as cold salad greens—can cause dampness, especially if you're a Spleen type. Like mildew in your walls, continuous exposure to wet-producing foods "wets" your Spleen. It becomes bogged down and sluggish, and eventually impedes its ability to function properly.

In Reese's case, if she had continued the diet that she thought was so healthy for her, her Spleen Qi would have continued to weaken and she eventually would have developed Spleen Qi dampness. Her prematurely sagging facial muscles that were making her so unhappy would have gotten worse. It's likely that if she had waited a few more months to see me, she also would have been complaining about waking up with a puffy face and bags under her eyes. She also might have started to develop cellulite and notice sensitivity to pollen and other allergens she had never had before. Her struggle with weight loss eventually could have turned into weight gain, despite her "healthy" diet, and her ability to digest food could have deteriorated further.

The foundation of a diet that strengthens the Spleen includes warming and sweet-flavored foods. Foods that are considered warming include eggs, chicken, lamb, and lean beef, because they warm the body when they are eaten. The Spleen and Stomach are most active in the morning from 7 to 11, so starting your day with a warming Spleen breakfast is crucial.

Sweet is the Spleen's preferred taste, but don't confuse it with the sweet taste of sugar. It relates to the *natural* sweetness found in nature's food, such as certain fruits, grains, and root vegetables.

To be warm, however, food needs to be cooked. Cooked foods are easier to digest than raw foods. This is the principal reason why Reese's daily salad was actually working against her. Although Reese thought her low-fat diet was healthy, she wasn't eating the diet best for her Organ type—or her facial appearance. There is nothing wrong with the kinds of fruits and vegetables Reese was eating except that she was eating them cold. As a Spleen type, her Spleen was more sensitive to the effect they have on the body. She would have been better off eating a vegetable soup and steamed greens rather than a salad.

When I started working with Reese, I recommended that she begin her day with a poached egg over brown rice, and that she concentrate on eating cooked vegetables rather than cold salads. Ginger is considered a warming spice, so I recommended she warm her Spleen by drinking ginger tea between meals.

"Your Spleen is like the engine of your car," I told her. "When it's cold, it doesn't run properly. For optimal functioning, it needs to be warm."

Likewise, if you are a Spleen type, you should primarily eat cooked foods. All cooking methods are fine, with the exception of deep-frying, which is hard on the digestive tract. Though warm foods are preferred, room temperature is acceptable, but avoid cold foods as much as you can, especially in the winter months when a chill can set into the Spleen more easily. This means avoiding frozen desserts and cold beverages. If you do indulge in ice cream or a cold beer, for example, do so infrequently and in small amounts. Also, avoid foods that produce moisture, such as dairy products, especially cheese, butter, and milk. Take advantage of aromatic spices and condiments with sweet flavors, such as cinnamon, cloves, garlic, and ginger. They not only stimulate digestion, but also reduce the potential for Spleen dampness.

The Spleen functions optimally when food is eaten slowly and in small quantities. By eating the traditional three squares a day and going hungry between meals, Reese was taxing her Spleen. She would have done better by following the routine of diets that advocate smaller, more frequent meals throughout the day.

It is important for everyone, but Spleen types in particular, to chew food slowly and completely, with intent on flavor. The time to stop eating is when you're satisfied, not when you're full.

When Reese changed her eating habits, she began to notice a difference in the way she felt within days. Her complexion began to clear, her digestion improved, and her energy increased. The fog that interfered with her concentration started to dissipate. After a few acupuncture treatments, her cheeks were less droopy and her jawline was more firm.

Reese's diet didn't require major adjustments, but the changes she made had a major impact on how she looked and felt. With weekly acupuncture treatments, acupressure instructions to do at home, and a few skin care tips, Reese's cheek muscles lifted, her blemishes disappeared, and the baggy cheeks she disliked so much diminished. After ten treatments, she was thrilled with the results.

The basics of a Spleen-strengthening diet are:

- Eat cooked foods rather than raw.
- Eat meals warm or at room temperature.

- Eat small, frequent meals.
- Avoid frozen foods, cold foods, and cold beverages.
- Avoid dairy products that come from cow's milk.

Foods That Complement a Healthy Spleen

To correct a sluggish Spleen and help lift saggy cheeks and improve muscle tone, focus your diet on these foods and this eating style that nourishes the Spleen. Get these foods in your daily diet as much as possible. The Three-Day Spleen Menu, including the Rejuvenating Recipes, takes advantage of the foods and ingredients that complement the Spleen.

FISH, FOWL, MEAT

When choosing animal and fish protein, be partial to these foods:

- Anchovies (canned or fresh)
- Beef (lean)
- Chicken (all parts)
- Chicken eggs
- Duck (in small portions)
- Goose (in small portions)
- Herring
- Lamb (all parts)
- Pork
- Rabbit
- Salmon (wild)
- Shrimp
- Turkey (all parts)
- White fish (catfish, cod, flounder, perch)

VEGETABLES

For many people, the hardest part of a Spleen diet is getting accustomed to eating vegetables cooked rather than raw. However, most of the vegetables that complement the Spleen are best cooked. They are:

- Cabbage
- Carrots
- Fennel
- Leeks
- Mushrooms
- Onions

- Potatoes
- Root vegetables (all roots, including parsnips, rutabaga, sweet potatoes, white potatoes, turnips, and yams)
- Scallions
- Snap peas
- String beans
- Winter squash (acorn, butternut, spaghetti)

FRUIT

Eating fruit is fine. The caveat is to eat it warm, meaning it should be poached or stewed. Fruits that are particularly Spleen friendly are:

- Apples
- Apricots
- Cherries
- Dates
- Figs
- Mangos
- Papaya
- Raspberries
- Strawberries

GRAINS

Whole grains are great, as long as you eat them cooked. That means avoiding cold cereals for breakfast. You can make breakfast cereals out of these grains in advance and heat them up in the microwave in the morning. A few morning cereal recipes are offered to get you started.

- Buckwheat
- Corn
- Millet
- Oats
- Rice (brown, glutinous, sweet, white)
- Whole wheat flour

LEGUMES

Legumes are hard to digest, and there are few that are good for the Spleen. When you want legumes, go for:

- Garbanzo beans (chickpeas)
- Kidney beans
- Peanuts
- Peas
- Yellow soybeans

NUTS AND SEEDS

Nuts and seeds as snacks and toppings are not Spleen foods, except for these two notables, which should be cooked and eaten in moderation:

- Chestnuts
- Peanuts

OILS/BUTTER

Regular butter and margarine you find in the market aren't part of a Spleen diet. However, these healthy and tasty oils are:

- Olive oil
- Safflower oil
- Sesame oil

BEVERAGES

If you are a soda or juice junkie, it may be a hard habit to break, but give it a try. Your Spleen will be forever grateful. The Spleen works well with:

- Warm (not iced) tea, especially ginger tea
- Wine (in moderation)

CONDIMENTS AND SPICES

Keep these condiments and spices in your cupboard, and rely on them in your recipes as much as possible. You can use them in all their forms:

- Agave nectar
- Basil
- Bay leaf
- Brown sugar (in small amounts)
- Caraway seeds
- Cardamom
- Chiles
- Chives
- Cilantro
- Cinnamon
- Cloves
- Garlic
- Ginger
- Honey
- Maple syrup
- Molasses

- Mustard
- Nutmeg
- Orange peel

- Pepper (black, cayenne, and white)
- Saffron

The Three-Day Spleen Diet

This is a sample of what a typical Spleen diet looks like. It is important to keep your meals small. Eating less food more frequently is better than three squares a day. If snacking is not your cup of tea, consider dividing your breakfast or lunch into two and eating half later in the day. Keep your dinner small and eat it several hours before bedtime.

DAY 1

BREAKFAST
Hot oatmeal with cinnamon and brown sugar

SNACK
Slice of rice toast with room-temperature hummus
Ginger tea

LUNCH
Warmed Leftovers and Rice Salad (page 103)

DINNER
Simmering Salmon with Asian Orange Sauce (page 103)
Steamed string beans
Baked white potato

SNACK
Baked apple

DAY 2

BREAKFAST
Rice Cream (page 101) with Mediterranean Stewed Fruit (page 102)

SNACK
Oat bran muffin
Ginger tea

LUNCH
Grilled shrimp
Braised Leeks (page 104)
Steamed white rice

DINNER
Mexican Lamb Patties (page 105)
Mashed Medley with Aromatic Spices (page 106)
Steamed fennel

DAY 3

BREAKFAST
Soft-boiled egg
Rice toast with safflower butter

SNACK
Honey-Nut Dates (page 107)
Ginger tea

LUNCH
Chunky Chicken Soup (page 105)

SNACK
Toasted rice bread

DINNER
Corn and kidney bean taco
Steamed vegetables (snap peas, mushrooms, scallions)
Perky Peaches with Berries (page 107)
Ginger tea

Rejuvenating Recipes

These Spleen-friendly recipes will give your taste buds and your face a lift!

RICE CREAM

Get a warm start on the day with this make-ahead breakfast. Creamy as oatmeal, it is the Spleen's answer to commercial cold cereals. Double the batch and it will last for the work week. Keep refrigerated and warm a serving by zapping it in the microwave.

> ½ cup uncooked brown rice
> 4 cups water
> Sea salt and freshly ground black pepper
> 1 tablespoon maple syrup or agave nectar

1   Place the rice and water in a medium saucepan, place over medium heat, and bring to a boil. Reduce the heat to the lowest setting and season with salt and pepper. Cover and cook for 1½ hours, or until the rice is very soft and the mixture looks like thick oatmeal when stirred.

2   Place the rice mixture, half at a time, in a blender and blend on low speed until smooth. Stir in the maple syrup. Serve hot.

MAKES 2 CUPS

MEDITERRANEAN STEWED FRUIT

This sweet treat is quite versatile. Serve it over hot oatmeal, as an accent to poultry, or as a stand-alone dessert or snack.

> ½ cup dried cherries
> ½ cup dried dates
> ½ cup dried figs
> ½ cup dried apricots
> ½ cup honey
> ¼ teaspoon ground cinnamon or nutmeg

Place the dried fruit in a large saucepan and cover with water. Place over medium heat, bring to a simmer, and stir in the honey. Cover and simmer until the fruit is tender, about 10 minutes. Sprinkle with cinnamon or nutmeg and serve warm.

SERVES 4

▨ SIMMERING SALMON WITH ASIAN ORANGE SAUCE

If possible, buy wild Alaskan sockeye salmon—not only is it tastier, but wild salmon is healthier than farm-raised salmon and is higher in omega-3 fatty acids.

4 4- to 6-ounce wild Alaskan sockeye salmon steaks
3 tablespoons sesame oil
2 tablespoons safflower butter or oil
1 teaspoon orange zest
Juice of ½ small orange
Juice of 1 medium lemon
Sea salt and freshly ground black pepper

1 Rinse the salmon steaks and pat dry. Heat the sesame oil over medium-high heat in a medium pan and brown the salmon steaks for 2 minutes on each side. Remove from the pan and transfer to a plate.

2 Add the safflower butter or oil to the same pan over low heat and warm it. Add the orange zest, orange juice, and lemon juice. Simmer for 2 minutes.

3 Return the salmon steaks to the pan and cook, turning them over a few times, until they are done to your liking. Season with salt and pepper.

SERVES 4

▨ WARMED LEFTOVERS AND RICE SALAD

This meal-in-one salad is a warm, filling way to enjoy your leftovers.

2 cups cubed leftover beef, pork, or chicken
2 cups water
1 cup uncooked brown rice
1 tablespoon extra virgin olive oil
1 cup sliced fresh mushrooms
1 15-ounce can peas, drained and rinsed
1 15-ounce can garbanzo beans, drained and rinsed
3 scallions, thinly sliced

3 garlic cloves, minced
Sea salt and freshly ground black pepper

1 Coarsely cube the leftover beef, pork, or chicken and put it in a medium bowl. Bring it to room temperature.

2 Bring the water to a boil in a medium saucepan. Add the rice, cover, and reduce the heat to low. Simmer for about 50 minutes, until the water is completely absorbed and the rice is soft. Do not stir while the rice is cooking. Set aside.

2 Heat the oil in a medium skillet over medium-high heat. Add the mushrooms and sauté about 3 minutes, or until tender. Add the peas, garbanzo beans, scallions, and garlic, lower the heat, and cook until warmed through, about 3 minutes.

4 Combine the warm vegetables, rice, and leftovers and mix gently. Season with salt and pepper. Serve warm or at room temperature.

SERVES 4

▦ BRAISED LEEKS

Follow the same recipe using Vidalia onions to make a topping for burgers.

½ teaspoon safflower oil
2 pounds leeks, trimmed, washed, and quartered lengthwise
1 cup chicken broth
1 tablespoon brown sugar

1 Heat the oil in a medium skillet over medium heat. Add the leeks and sauté lightly, about 1 minute.

2 Add the chicken broth and bring to a simmer. Cover and braise, stirring occasionally, until the leeks are slightly tender, about 12 minutes. Remove the lid and cook for another 10 minutes, or until the broth has almost evaporated.

3 Increase the heat to high and sprinkle the brown sugar over the leeks. Cook, stirring frequently, for another 10 minutes, or until the leeks are lightly caramelized.

SERVES 4

▥ CHUNKY CHICKEN SOUP

A soup you eat with a knife and fork. Great for a Sunday supper.

> 1 whole chicken, about 3 pounds
> 4 carrots, peeled and cut into large chunks
> 4 celery stalks, trimmed and cut in half
> 2 parsnips, peeled and cut into large chunks
> 2 medium potatoes, cut in half
> 2 leeks, trimmed and cut in half
> 1 large onion, peeled and quartered
> 1 whole garlic clove, smashed
> 1 large slice green pepper
> 1 parsley sprig
> Sea salt and freshly ground black pepper

1 Put the chicken in a large pot and cover completely with water. Add the remaining ingredients and bring to a low boil. Reduce the heat and simmer, uncovered, until the chicken meat starts to fall off the bones, about 3 hours.

2 Discard the garlic clove, green pepper slice, and parsley sprig. Divide the chicken pieces and vegetables among 4 bowls. Spoon the broth on top and serve.

SERVES 4

▥ MEXICAN LAMB PATTIES

> 1 pound lean ground lamb
> 6 fresh chives, minced
> 3 garlic cloves, minced
> 2 tablespoons ground cumin
> 2 scallions, chopped
> 2 tablespoons minced parsley or mint
> 1 tablespoon safflower butter or oil
> Juice of 1 medium lemon
> Sea salt and freshly ground black pepper

1 Put the ground lamb in a large bowl and add the chives, garlic, cumin, scallions, and mint. Mix well. Mold into 4 large patties.

2 In a large skillet, brown the safflower butter over medium heat. Add the patties and cook for 3 minutes on each side. Continue cooking for 5 minutes, turning occasionally. Test one patty with a sharp knife. The patty should be pink in the center. Remove the patties, add the lemon juice to the pan drippings, and pour over the patties. Season with salt and pepper.

SERVES 4

MASHED MEDLEY WITH AROMATIC SPICES

The spices bring the flavor of the Far East to these warming winter root vegetables.

I turnip, peeled and quartered
I acorn squash, quartered
I sweet potato or yam, quartered
½ tablespoon safflower oil
I ½ teaspoons ground nutmeg
I teaspoon ground cardamom
½ teaspoon ground cloves
I tablespoon honey
Sea salt and freshly ground black pepper

I Put the turnip, squash, and potato or yam in a medium saucepan and cover with water. Bring to a boil, lower the heat, cover, and cook until all of the vegetables are tender, about 20 minutes. Drain, saving ½ cup of the cooking water. Let the vegetables sit until cool enough to handle.

2 Peel the vegetables, place them in a medium bowl, and mash, adding the reserved water by the tablespoon until the puree reaches a smooth consistency.

3 Heat the oil on medium to high heat in a small heavy skillet, preferably cast-iron. Add the nutmeg, cardamom, and cloves, blend in the honey, and stir for about I minute, until they release their aroma. Stir into the mashed vegetables and season with salt and pepper.

SERVES 4

▦ HONEY-NUT DATES

A nutritious snack or dessert.

> 12 fresh or dried dates, pitted
> 12 cooked chestnuts
> 2 egg yolks
> 1 teaspoon honey
> ¼ teaspoon orange zest
> 12 strips orange zest

1 Slice the dates in half. Insert 1 chestnut into each half and then place in a serving dish.

2 In a medium bowl, beat the egg yolks* until fluffy, then add the honey and orange zest. Drizzle over the dates. Twist the orange peel to form curlicues and garnish each date with a twist.

> * *Warning:* Consuming raw and lightly cooked eggs may carry the slight risk of salmonella or other food-borne illness. To reduce this risk, use only fresh, properly refrigerated, clean grade A or AA eggs with intact shells.

MAKES 24 PIECES

▦ PERKY PEACHES WITH BERRIES

This is a satisfying warm dessert and a great way for Spleen types to enjoy peaches in season. You can make it ahead and refrigerate, but bring it to room temperature before serving.

> 2 tablespoons honey
> 2 fresh ripe peaches, halved and pitted
> 5 strawberries, hulled
> 3 tablespoons molasses
> ½ cup blueberries
> Fresh mint sprigs, for garnish

1 Fill a shallow pan, one large enough to accommodate the peaches in one layer, with water. Bring the water to a simmer over medium heat. Stir in the honey.

Gently add the peach halves to the water with a spoon. Simmer, uncovered, for 5 minutes. Remove the peaches and set aside.

2 Put the strawberries and molasses in the bowl of a blender and blend until smooth. Spoon the strawberry puree over the peach halves. Sprinkle with blueberries and decorate with mint sprigs.

MAKES 4 SERVINGS

How to Give Your Face Extra Lift

When women take their sagging Spleen faces to the spa, estheticians treat them to a facial made up of expensive products, such as lifting and tightening skin creams and masks. Face masks are an important part of any skin care regimen, but for Spleen types prone to sagging cheek muscles, they are most important. And you should get one more frequently than during an occasional trip to the spa. Spleen types should treat themselves to a mask once a week.

Facial masks sound luxurious, but they don't have to be expensive. In fact, you can give yourself a spa face mask with ingredients found right in your kitchen. The foods that belong in a Spleen-friendly diet are so versatile you can even wear many of them! These at-home masks are inexpensive, natural, and easy to assemble. Most important, you'll find they are quite effective. Increase or decrease the ingredient proportions to suit your desired consistency or result. Before using any product, whether homemade or purchased, I recommend performing a skin allergy patch test (page 219).

EGG-ON-YOUR-FACE INSTANT LIFT

Egg white is especially useful for tightening the skin, so Spleen types should take advantage of this easy-to-use beauty aid. Albumin, the protein found in egg whites, is well known among major cosmetics companies for toning and firming the skin. In addition, egg whites help reduce the appearance of large or uneven pores to give you that smooth-looking glow. For an instant facelift for sagging skin, all you need is to break an egg, separate the white from the yolk, and apply the egg white as a mask! Leave it on for fifteen minutes, then wash it off with warm water. Many women swear by it for giving them a "Cinderella moment"—right before a special occasion or special night out when they want their skin to look its best.

▓ LEMON LIFT

This recipe, with a boost of refreshing lemon, is great for a puffy face and an oily complexion, and it will make your skin feel toned, tight, and taut.

> 1 egg white
> ⅓ teaspoon lemon juice

Combine the egg white with the lemon juice and apply to your face, being careful to stay away from your eyes. Relax and let it set in for 15 minutes. Rinse off with warm water. Apply weekly or as desired.

▓ KIWI QUICKIE FACE MASK

The benefits of kiwi are very similar to those of lemon. Both tone and brighten dull skin and give you a smooth, radiant appearance. The honey acts as a moisturizer and antibacterial, which means it also helps get rid of breakouts.

> 1 ripe kiwi, peeled
> ½ teaspoon honey

1 Blend the kiwi in a blender or mash with a fork if it is soft. Strain the juice from the pulp. Discard the juice or save it for another use.

2 Using a fork, combine the pulp with the honey. Apply the mask to your face, being careful to avoid the eye area. Leave the mask on for 15 minutes. Rinse off with warm water. Apply weekly or as desired.

▓ FIRMING MASK FOR SAGGING FACE

This is a great treatment for tired, sagging face muscles and puffy eyes. While you are relaxing with the mask on your face, you should feel its tightening effect and the soothing effect of the tea bags on your eyes. This treatment will leave you with your face feeling lifted and rejuvenated.

> 2 black tea bags
> 1 tablespoon minced carrot
> 1 large egg white
> 1 teaspoon coconut oil (cooking oil)
> 1 teaspoon honey
> ½ teaspoon ground ginger
> 1 large piece of gauze cut to the size of your face

1 Soak the tea bags in warm water for 20 minutes. Meanwhile, steam or cook the minced carrots in a little boiling water until they are very soft, about 10 minutes. Set aside to cool.

2 Beat the egg white in a small bowl until frothy. Add the carrot, coconut oil, honey, and ginger and mix well with a fork until the mixture has a smooth consistency.

3 Cut holes in the gauze for your eyes and nostrils. Place the gauze in the mixture and let it soak for about 1 minute, until the gauze is saturated with the mixture. Remove and gently squeeze excess moisture from the gauze with your fingertips.

4 Remove the tea bags from the water and squeeze out the excess moisture with your fingertips. Lie down in a comfortable position and apply the gauze to your face. Close your eyes and place the tea bags over your eyelids. Relax for 15 minutes.

5 Remove the tea bags and mask. Rinse your face well with warm water, followed by cool water, with your hands or a soft washcloth. Apply your favorite moisturizing cream.

▨ BRUISING MASK

Arnica is a homeopathic remedy for bruising and swelling. When combined with cayenne pepper it quickly penetrates through the skin surface, improving circulation and reducing healing time.

5 teaspoons arnica cream
1 teaspoon safflower oil
½ teaspoon cayenne pepper

Put the arnica cream is a small clean bowl or jar and mix in the oil and cayenne. Rub it into the affected area two or three times a day until the bruise disappears. Apply weekly or as desired. *Avoid direct eye contact.*

IF YOU DON'T WANT TO MAKE IT, THEN BUY IT . . .

Neal's Yard Remedies Rejuvenating Frankincense Firming Mask

Cost: About $40

Size: 50 ml

This product is made with frankincense, a resin collected from the bark of the frankincense tree. It is reputed to have regenerative, anti-aging, and hydrating powers. This mask is designed to firm, lift, brighten, and soothe all types of skin. You can see and feel the difference.

Nefeli Facial Rejuvenating Mask

Cost: About $65

Size: 4 packages

Made with three Chinese herbs—angelica, safflower, and ginseng—this facial rejuvenating mask lifts, firms, and diminishes the appearance of sagging, bags, fine lines, and wrinkles. Angelica helps improve blood circulation, safflower replenishes moisture, and ginseng rejuvenates and stimulates the production of youthful-looking skin.

Origins Youthtopia Firming Eye Cream with Rhodiola

Cost: About $43

Size: .5 oz.

This is a fast-absorbing eye cream that acts like a mask. *Rhodiola rosea*, an antioxidant-rich flowering herb, and amalaki, a vitamin C–rich berry, are the key ingredients in this formula. When combined they help lift, hydrate, and firm the delicate skin under your eyes without drying it out.

7

Dry and Withered Skin: Nourishing the Lungs

WHEN JOHN, AGE FORTY-THREE, CAME INTO MY office, his face looked pale and his skin tone was dull and dry. I could tell right away by the way he lethargically shuffled into the room and sank into the chair that he had a Qi deficiency. As we talked, I noticed he sighed a lot. When I asked him about it, he said he sometimes felt like he wasn't getting enough air.

Physically, he was tall and trim with angular, birdlike features—pointy nose, chin, and ears. I was not surprised to learn that he was an avid runner. What struck me the most about him was his voice—soft and whispery. I continuously found myself having to ask him to repeat himself.

John didn't come to see me only because he was concerned about his appearance; he was more worried about the way he felt. Although he wasn't youth-obsessed, he couldn't help noticing how pale and drawn he had become. He had always loved going for long jogs after work and on weekends, but the pleasure it used to give him had disappeared.

"I don't feel good about myself," he sighed. "I used to take pride in myself and my life. My girlfriend says that I've become aloof and distant, but that's not really what's going on. I just don't seem to care much about anything."

During one of John's breathless pauses, I asked him when this all began. He responded by saying, "My best friend passed away in August, and about two months later I got really sick. It lasted for a while, probably several months. At first I thought it was just a cold; I often get colds in the fall. But then it went into my throat and chest. No fever or congestion, just a dry cough. I also feel weak and tired."

John said he has always believed in natural medicine, but his girlfriend was skeptical. "She made me promise to see a 'real' doctor, which I did. He gave me antibiotics. I had to take several rounds before I started to feel better. My illness went away, but I feel as if I never really recovered. I thought some acupuncture might help. That's why I'm here." Then he whispered behind a cupped hand, "Even though my girlfriend doesn't know yet."

At this point it was clear that the grief of losing his best friend, in addition to his long-standing illness, resulted in John's Lung Qi deficiency. Grief caused by an upheaval in life, such as the death of a loved one, can really take a toll on Lung types like John. To confirm my diagnosis, I took a look at his hands. I couldn't help but notice that the hairs on the back of his hands looked thin and patchy.

"Your hands are dry and you have a rash on your fingers," I said. "Did this develop after the loss of your friend as well?" I also asked him if he had been unusually susceptible to colds over the winter. "Constipation a problem, too?" Yes, yes, and yes were his answers.

I told John a series of acupuncture treatments to get his Lung Qi flowing and attention to his diet would get him feeling much better. I didn't say a word about what it would do for his complexion. It was a surprise I was going to let him discover for himself.

Eight weeks of treatments and getting more dairy foods, whole grain rice, and vegetables into his diet produced a profound change in John, both mentally and physically. Emotionally, he still missed his friend, but he no longer felt forlorn. Physically, he stopped coughing, felt stronger, his energy level improved, and he even started to enjoy running again. His skin regained its moisture, his rash disappeared, and his complexion returned to its rosy glow. Also, his voice was noticeably stronger. Jokingly, he said that his girlfriend finally understood him!

Complementary Organ: Large Intestine

Primary function: Maintaining healthy skin and body hair

Facial concern: Dry, oily, or problem skin

Emotional regulation: Grief

Complementary orifice: Nose

Season: Fall

Color: White

Taste: Spicy

Primary evil: Dryness

Active time: 3 a.m. to 7 a.m.

"My complexion is the envy of my girlfriend, because hers hasn't been looking too good lately," he said. "She's unhappy about her skin and she's having a lot of skin problems. I think she's going to come see you about a rejuvenating treatment."

Sure enough, a few weeks later I was sitting with John's girlfriend, Sandy, explaining Acu-Facial® acupuncture and acupressure. Organized with pen in hand, she came with a list of questions and concerns about her condition. Ever the skeptic!

I found it remarkable how John and Sandy were so similar in their physique. She, too, at forty years of age, was tall and thin with a long, narrow face. However, unlike John's dull and dry skin, hers was oily and blemished. When we got to the subject of diet, she got flustered. "I eat healthy, but now, no matter how much fiber I eat, it seems like I'm always having trouble with constipation," she said.

She, too, had been ill over the winter. She figured she got it from John, but instead of feeling weak and tired like John, she described her symptoms as flushed and feverish. Her doctor also gave her antibiotics, which improved her condition, but her normally healthy, flawless skin had taken a turn for the worse. "I don't understand this," she said. "I wash my face morning and night. I use the best products. I don't drink alcohol and I mostly eat fresh, organic food. This shouldn't be happening to me."

Her true emotional side started to show when we talked about John's deceased best friend. Although she liked him a lot, she had known him only since after she met John, so she said she did not experience the same depth of sadness as John did. She felt her boyfriend's pain and tried to be compassionate. "Expressing my feelings is not my strength," she said. "I have a tendency to intellectualize them. I try not to judge John for taking it so hard for so long, but sometimes I can't help myself. I'm really not a mean person, I just want things to be the same as they were before this happened."

I carefully explained that from an Eastern medicine point of view, even though their symptoms were different, she, too, was a Lung type and susceptible to a Lung deficiency. John's emotional pain and prolonged illness had created a weakness in his Lung Qi. With Sandy it was a little different. Her Lungs were exhibiting signs of the Chinese evil heat, which most likely caused her physical illness. I explained the facial changes she was experiencing had a direct relationship to the heat in her Lungs.

Because she was unfamiliar with Eastern medicine, I could tell that Sandy was not a hundred percent trusting of my explanation. "Let's give acupuncture a try," I said. "You saw how much it helped John. I believe it will help you, too." Though still skeptical, Sandy committed to acupuncture for a month. After two treatments, and remarkable results, she signed up for an additional month. At this point, I recommended a few skin care changes. After eight treatments, her once flawless skin was again healthy and blemish-free, and her bowels were back to normal.

Profile of a Lung Type

Lung types are generally small-boned and angular with soft, prominent features and small, trim, compact muscles. When their Lungs are healthy, their skin radiates a smooth and healthy glow that is the envy of others. This is due to their small and even skin pores—nature's intended design.

Lung types are fastidious and well organized, from the way they dress to the way they speak. Keeping order in their lives is paramount. They believe there is a place for everything, and they keep everything in place. This neat and kempt appearance transcends to other aspects of life. They are honest and fair to the point that they are extremely sensitive, though they keep their emotions to themselves. They are so calm and composed that they often come across as emotionally distant. Truth be known, they are emotionally fragile to the point that it can negatively influence their Lung Qi.

Lung types strive for perfection, crave structure, and are most comfortable in situations in which they know the rules and follow them exactly. They succeed by adhering to the order of their lives. They live according to a personal set of principles and ruffle easily when their order is threatened. As a result, they respond poorly to change. They often get flustered when situations appear "out of control."

For Lung types, getting out of their comfort zone is like trying to cruise in traffic with the hand brake engaged. It causes Lung Qi to sputter and lose its drive. When the Lungs get out of balance it is reflected in the pores, which get too small to properly make or draw in moisture, or too large so that too much escapes. Both produce dramatic changes in the skin, hair, nails, and mucous membranes.

When pores get too small, it usually shows up as excessive dryness, such as brittle nails and dry skin. Body hair loses its moisture as well, something men notice most in the texture of their beard. Less often, it is just the opposite—oily skin and hair—as a result of the pores enlarging. Either way, a break in the delicate chemistry of the pores can cause a rash of health problems, which is why Lung types are prone to skin problems and other illnesses. Skin irritations, such as rashes, eczema, psoriasis, rosacea, and sweating problems, either too much or too little, are common. They are also prone to respiratory problems, such as asthma, colds, flu, sinus problems, allergies, and congestion in their nose, throat, and sinuses. Face and body hair can become thin or patchy. They are also sensitive to temperature change and commonly complain about having cold hands and feet. Alternatively, pore size can swell and their skin becomes oily and blemished.

When the Lungs are weak, Qi isn't strong enough to assist their complementary Organ, the Large Intestine, with proper elimination. As a result, this causes constipation, diarrhea, or other bowel problems.

When Lung types get out of balance, you can see it in their personality, as their need to maintain order intensifies. Critical thoughts and judgmental behavior compensate for their inner feelings of self-doubt, ambivalence, and confusion. Like Sandy, they can become rigid, indifferent, and aloof. As in the case of John, they can even sink into unshakable sadness and grief.

Need for Control a Common Trait

Inhale, exhale. Breathing gives us the ability to sustain life. It represents the Lungs' ability to govern the experience of living and feeling one moment, one step, one day at a time.

Have you ever noticed that when you try to prevent yourself from crying, you stop breathing? When sadness or grief overwhelm, there is a tendency to try to cut yourself off from your feelings by holding your breath. When your Lung Qi is strong, you are able to breathe with and experience your feelings without resisting them. Breathing with healthy Lung Qi allows your chest and diaphragm to expand, your shoulders to open, and your chin, head, and face to lift.

Repression of or too much sadness and grief can hurt your Lungs. It causes your rib cage to drop, your chest to sink, and your chin and head to droop downward. When your posture collapses, it further decreases the ability of your Lungs to circulate Qi, mist your skin, and experience emotion.

The Lungs govern the desire for structure and boundaries, so a Lung type's personality is also well defined and structured. Psychologically, Sandy was the typical Lung type. In our initial visit she arrived with a list of questions. Neatly dressed, she sat with poised posture, pen and pad in hand. She listened intently, took notes, and often repeated my answers for clarification. Although she came for acupuncture treatment, she first needed to understand what was about to happen to her. Unlike Spleen-type Reese's trusting, bubbly personality, Sandy was contained and controlled. She kept her emotions in check and intellectualized her feelings.

The Role of the Lungs for Healthy Skin

Healthy Lungs are personified in glowing skin, due to the Lungs' primary responsibility, which is to nourish and maintain healthy pore size, skin, and proper breathing.

Western medicine views the lungs solely as a vital organ responsible for the respiratory system—our ability to take air into the lungs through the mouth and nose and expel carbon dioxide. Eastern medicine has a more expansive concept of the role of this vital Organ. It sees the Lungs as responsible for all parts of the body that "breathe." This includes the skin, the largest organ of the body, with pores that cover us from head to toe.

This means that when your Lungs are healthy, your skin is soft and dewy and your pore size is even. When your Lungs are weak, your skin changes in texture and quality. It can become thick or thin, dull or blemished, dry or oily. Damage to your Lungs can occur in many ways. Weather conditions, especially overexposure to wind, cold, and heat, affects the Lungs. Lung damage is common among people who live in perpetually dry climates, such as Arizona, New Mexico, and other desert-like areas of the western United States, such as parts of Southern California. Excessive sadness or grief, due to the combination of emotional turmoil and too many tears, affects the Lungs and can have a profound impact on Lung types, as it did with John.

As with all Organs, an imbalance in another Organ can impact the Lungs. Spleen dampness or Kidney weakness are the conditions most likely to interfere with Lung Qi. By the same token, a weakness in the Lungs can negatively impact the Large Intestine, which is why Lung types are prone to bowel problems.

Only Normal Skin Is Normal

Western medicine and Eastern medicine have quite different takes on what it means to have healthy skin. Western specialists believe we are all born with a skin *type*—normal, oily, dry, a combination of oily and dry, or sensitive. It is yours for life and generally does not change much. Westerners believe it is perfectly natural for the quality of the skin to vary from one person to the next.

Western medicine also says that certain skin types are prone to certain skin *conditions*. This includes a long list of problems, ranging from acute outbreaks of rashes or acne to chronic skin conditions, such as eczema and psoriasis.

Eastern medicine sees it differently. Chinese doctrine says we are all born with normal skin. When skin becomes oily, dry, or a combination of both, or is sensitive, it isn't because it's our destiny or the result of a skin condition we somehow "pick up." If the feel of the skin and the look of the pores are anything but normal, this is most likely due to a Lung Qi imbalance.

There are many outside factors that affect Lung Qi and show up as problem skin or changes in the texture of the skin. Among them are environmental conditions, such as weather changes or pollution; an excessive lifestyle, such as a poor diet or too much drinking; fluctuating hormones, especially around menstruation; taking certain medications; the state of your health; aging; and your daily skin care habits. I discuss these influences, as well as skin types, in more detail in Chapter 11.

How the Lungs Function

The Lungs work closely with the Spleen. After receiving food nutrients from the Spleen, your Lungs mix them with the air you breathe to create healthy Qi. It then sends the healthy Qi to the rest of the Organs and throughout the entire body. The remaining impure Qi is expelled through your nose, your pores, and Large Intestine.

When you have a Lung imbalance, it means your Lungs are too weak to create enough Qi. The quality of the Qi and the Lungs' ability to distribute it is compromised as well. Like a plant without water, an insufficiency of Qi in your skin causes your skin and pores to become dry and withered. Without enough Qi, your other Organs and Meridians become weak, too. John's pale complexion, dry, dull skin tone, and fatigue were caused by his weak Lung Qi. I used acupuncture on the Meridian pathways to the Lungs and Large Intestine to strengthen them, so they could distribute healthy Qi.

Moisture: A Delicate Balance

In addition to the creation and distribution of Qi, the Lungs regulate internal water flow by turning some of the Qi into moisture. After receiving nutrients from the Spleen, the Lungs transform this form of Qi into a fine mist that permeates your body from head to toe, inward toward the center of your body and outward to the surface of your skin, much like a sprinkler nurtures a lawn. It produces the soft, dewy, and lustrous appearance that your skin craves—all the result of healthy water flow expelled from your Lungs.

The Lungs need to stay moist in order to spread healthy Qi to other parts of the body and mist your skin properly—not too much, not too little. This is why people who live in dry climates are prone to Lung damage. However, it can also be a problem for people in cold climates who are exposed to dry heat in the home or office. Even overexposure to the cozy blaze of a fireplace can be harmful to the Lungs. Dry heat interferes with the Lungs' ability to do their job.

There is, however, an instance when moisture creates a problem. Because the Lungs are so dependent on the Spleen, the health of your Spleen affects the health of your Lungs. When your Spleen gets damp, its ability to sort nutrients properly becomes impaired. Instead of sending unhealthy nutrients down to the Stomach for digestion and elimination, it sends them upward to the Lungs. Like a clogged drain, the Lungs get congested and can no longer sort and mist effectively. When this happens, the Lungs can also get backed up and they, too, become damp. When dampness in the Lungs lingers, the moisture begins to heat and swell, like bread rising. With no place to go, it tries to push itself outward through the surface of your face and body.

The primary areas of elimination are through your nose, skin, and Large Intestine. When damp heat escapes, your nose gets dry and your skin dries, gets irritated, and can break out in pimples. You can also get constipated. That's what happened to Sandy. Her oily, irritated, blemished skin, dry nose, and constipation were due to damp heat exiting her body.

The Lungs and the Six Evils

The primary evil associated with the Lungs is dryness, though this Organ is susceptible to all the evils. Exposure to arid conditions, such as living in the desert or sitting in front of a fireplace, eating too much spicy food, and drinking too much alcohol can make the Lungs dry. When this happens, the Lungs lose some of their ability to send air throughout the body. Dry skin, nostrils, and lips, shortness of breath, and constipation are all signs of dryness harming the Lungs.

Wind can be a major problem for the Lungs. It can invade your Lungs on its own, but it likes to take other evils along for the ride. For example, wind can carry cold or heat from the outside environment through your skin and into your body. This means that if you are a Lung type, you have a lot working against you!

What is commonly referred to as cold in Western medicine is called wind invasion in Chinese medicine. Wind commonly invades the body

CHARACTERISTICS OF A LUNG TYPE

Signs of healthy Lungs are:

- Delicate, soft, smooth skin
- Even pore size
- Small bones, delicate features, compact muscles
- Healthy immune system
- Fastidious appearance
- Highly organized habits and skills
- Composed behavior
- Honesty, fairness, and the aim for perfection

Signs of unhealthy Lungs are:

- Poor skin quality
- Pores that are too large or too small
- Excessive oily or dry skin
- Chronic nasal congestion or dryness
- Susceptibility to colds or flu
- Chronic breathing problems, such as shortness of breath or asthma
- Blotchy face and patchy body hair
- Frequent constipation
- Rigid behavior, judgmental thoughts
- Chronic sadness or prolonged grief

through the skin. Have you ever noticed how different you look when you feel sick? When your Lungs are not functioning properly, they lose their ability to control the strength of your pores, especially on the face and the hair follicles beneath the skin of your body. This causes a weakening of the secure skin barrier that protects you against wind, cold, and heat. Without strong Lung Qi, you become defenseless, like a sorcerer without a wand. When a cold wind permeates your skin and settles in your body, it is called wind-cold. It makes you look puffy and pale, you feel stuffy in your nose and face, and you get the chills.

When wind carries heat into your body, it is called wind-heat. This is why on a blustery day your complexion gets flushed and your skin and the inside of your nose get dry. If your Lungs are relatively healthy, your complexion, skin, and nose will quickly return to normal. However, when you have a Lung Qi deficiency, instead of getting better, you begin to feel worse. It can leave you feeling headachy and feverish, and then you get sick.

Lung Qi is similar to the immune system. If your Lung Qi is strong, you can resist or quickly recover from the invasion of wind-cold or wind-heat. If your Lung Qi is compromised, then you can develop a cold or the flu. If you are a Lung type and you struggle with Lung Organ weakness, coming down with a simple cold or flu can lead to deeper problems, such as a chronic skin condition, frequent colds, respiratory problems, constipation, allergies, or even asthma. This is what happened to both John and Sandy.

Self-Acupressure for Improving Skin Tone

Anyone who has been to a dermatologist, has had a facial, or been to a beauty consultant knows their "skin type" and is advised how to take care of their skin accordingly. Eastern doctors believe we can all have normal skin. All it takes is good Lung Qi.

If you're unhappy with your skin tone or just want to restore a fresh-looking appearance to your face, follow this program. By applying acupressure to these points, you will help restore your Lung Qi and see a visible difference in your skin tone and appearance. You can use this regimen as a stand-alone treatment or integrate it into your AcuFacial® Acupressure Face-lift protocol. You should see and feel noticeable results within twenty days.

In this routine, you start with your legs, then move to your hands, elbows, and face. Do each massage three times on both sides of the body in a clockwise rotation for ten rotations before moving onto the next body part. Read the section "Touch and Go: Key Acupressure Points" on page 30 before beginning this routine.

LEGS

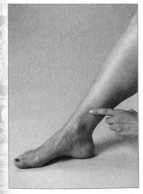

Spleen 6

Spleen 6 | SP 6 is located on the inside of the leg, roughly four finger-widths above the top of the ankle (medial) bone. It balances and strengthens the Qi and Blood of the Liver, Spleen, and Kidneys and helps give your skin a toned, youthful, and radiant glow.

Stomach 36 | Move up your legs to your knees. ST 36 is located in the depression four finger-widths below the bottom of your knee on the outside of the leg bone (fibula). This point lifts the cheek muscles, strengthens the digestive system, and improves immune function. It is also used to strengthen your protective Lung Qi.

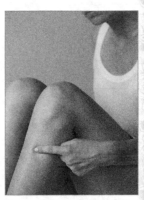

Stomach 36

HANDS

Lung 9 | Bend your wrist forward toward your inner arm. L 9 is located in the crease of your wrist, below the thumb, between the thumb bone and the tendon. This massage strengthens the Lungs and builds Lung Qi. It helps get rid of face puffiness.

Large Intestine 4 | Hold one hand out with your thumb resting beside your index finger. LI 4 is the soft spot between these two digits at the base of the thumb. Keep your hand in this position as you do the massage. This acupressure point sends Qi to the face and helps brighten the complexion.

ARMS

Large Intestine 11 | Bend your elbow into your body at a 90-degree angle. LI 11 is at the elbow, on the outside edge of the elbow crease. This acupressure point helps clear facial puffiness and nasal and sinus congestion.

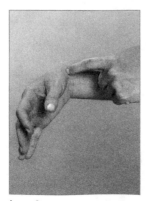

Lung 9

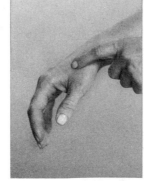

Large Intestine 4

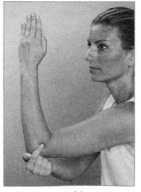

Large Intestine 11

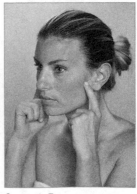

Triple Heater 17

NECK

Triple Heater 17 | TH 17 is located in the depression below the ears at the base of the skull. This is the primary lymphatic drainage point for the face. Massaging this pressure point reduces congestion, swelling, and puffiness in the face.

FACE

Large Intestine 20 | Move your fingers closer inward to the indentation right by the nostril and you will be on LI 20. This pressure point opens up and clears nasal congestion. Just as with ST 3, do this even if you don't feel congested.

Stomach 3 | ST 3 is located directly below the center of the eye at the level of the nostril. You can feel slight pressure in your sinus when you press it, and for good reason. This pressure point helps clear up sinus congestion. Even if you don't feel congested, massage this point as part of this routine.

Stomach 7 | ST 7 is located in front of your ear. You can find it by feeling for the depression between the cheekbone and the jawbone. It is used to lift the cheek muscles. This pressure point stimulates circulation in the face.

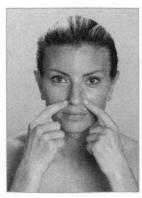

Large Intestine 20

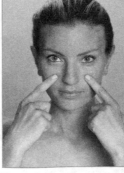

Stomach 3

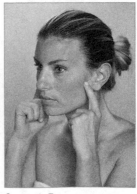

Stomach 7

9-1-1 HEALING THERAPY: COLDS AND FLU

The common cold and flu are the result of weak Lung Qi. If you are feverish, thirsty, sweaty, and have a sore throat, it is likely that they are being caused by wind-heat. If you have the chills, crave warmth, and have aches and pains all over, chances are you have wind-cold in your Lungs. Each takes a different dietary approach to strengthen Lung Qi.

Wind-Heat: Wind-heat is drying, so to counteract it, concentrate on eating foods that produce moisture. Grapefruit is a great healer for wind-heat in the Lungs. Other helpful foods are lemons, parsley, pears, peppermint, tofu, and turnips.

Wind-Cold: Spicy-hot foods are generally not for Lung types, except when the condition is wind-cold. Chicken soup is the classic home remedy for a cold and flu, but only if you have wind-cold rather than wind-heat. Truth is, any soup will help as long as it is hot and spicy. The best ingredients to spice up your soup are cayenne, garlic, scallions, and chili pepper. Eat soup often throughout the day. Also, sip plenty of ginger tea. To make ginger tea, steep 1 tablespoon of grated fresh ginger in one cup of boiled water for 5 minutes.

The pressure points to massage when you have a cold or the flu are those used to restore Lung Qi but should be followed in this order. Do the routine three times.

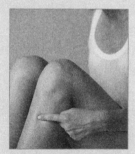

Stomach 36

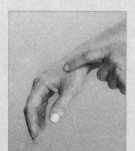

Large Intestine 4

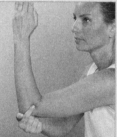

Large Intestine 11

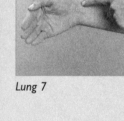

Lung 7

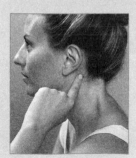

Triple Heater 17

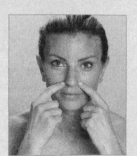

Large Intestine 20

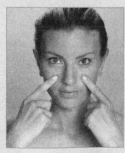

Stomach 3

Eating for Healthy Skin

There are only two goals when eating for healthy Lungs, and they are equally important: Eat from the bounty of moisture-producing foods, and avoid foods that will dry you out.

High on the list of moisture-producing foods are fresh vegetables and certain fruits and grains, because they contain so much water. If you've ever set string beans or watercress out in the hot sun, or left fresh vegetables in the refrigerator for too long, you've seen them shrivel up without the moisture your Lungs crave.

Protein is also important in maintaining strong Lung Qi. In fact, a craving for protein can be an indication of Lung Qi deficiency. The best protein for a Lung type is low fat, so stick with white meat, beans, and grains as much as possible.

Unless you have wind-cold in your Lungs, it is especially important to avoid foods and beverages that are drying and will rob your body of moisture. Avoid:

COLOR ME WHITE

If you're a Lung type, white should be your favorite color when it comes to food. To strengthen your Lungs, put these foods high on your list:

- Cauliflower
- Coconut
- Cucumber
- Lobster
- Lotus root
- Milk
- Mushrooms
- Onions
- Pears
- Potatoes
- Radishes
- Scallops
- Sesame seeds
- Tofu
- Turkey
- Water chestnuts
- White fish
- White radishes
- White rice
- White wine vinegar
- Yogurt

- Alcoholic beverages (although cooking with wine is okay because it acts as a carrier to expedite the effects of other ingredients)
- Coffee
- Caffeinated soft drinks
- Spicy foods

Also, keep in mind that Lung types are especially susceptible to the negative effects of cigarettes and recreational drugs.

Foods That Complement Healthy Lungs

FISH, FOWL, MEAT

Because Lung Qi depends on protein for nourishment, make sure to get some every day. The Lungs' preference for white foods is a reminder to keep it lean. When eating fowl, remove the skin. Protein foods that are Lung friendly include:

- Beef (keep portions small—no more than 4 ounces no more than two or three times a week)
- Chicken (all parts, skin removed)
- Duck breast
- Fish (all varieties of white fish)
- Goose (breast meat)
- Herring
- Mussels
- Rabbit (white meat)
- Turkey (all parts)

VEGETABLES

Though all vegetables are fair game for the Lungs because of their water content, these are considered the top picks:

- Asparagus
- Broccoli
- Carrots
- Cauliflower
- Celery
- Corn
- Cucumber
- Eggplant
- Leeks
- Lettuce
- Lotus root
- Mushrooms (white)
- Mustard greens
- Onions (all varieties)
- Potatoes (all varieties)
- Radishes (raw rather than cooked)
- Seaweed (especially kelp)
- Scallions
- Spinach
- Squash (all varieties)
- String beans
- Turnips
- Watercress (raw or steamed)
- Yams

FRUIT

Eat fruit raw rather than cooked to retain its moisture, and stay away from dried fruits.

- Apples
- Apricots (fresh only)
- Bananas
- Coconut
- Dates (red and black; fresh only)
- Grapefruit
- Grapes (all varieties)
- Lemons
- Longans
- Loquats
- Olives
- Oranges
- Peaches
- Pears (all varieties)
- Persimmons
- Raspberries
- Strawberries
- Tangerines

GRAINS

Grains are great for the Lungs because they bulk up with moisture as they cook. These are the grains most desired by the Lungs:

- Buckwheat
- Rye
- Rice (all colors and varieties)

LEGUMES

Legumes offer excellent fiber, which is important for the constipation that frequently accompanies a Lung Qi imbalance. Sprouted legumes and peanuts can be eaten raw, or choose from this list and cook them well:

- Kidney beans
- Tofu (baked, broiled, sautéed, or steamed)
- Soybeans

NUT AND SEEDS

Nuts and seeds make great snacks and offer nutrition, fiber, and protein to nourish the Lungs.

- Almonds
- Chestnuts (baked, boiled, or steamed)
- Pine nuts (raw)
- Sunflower seeds
- Walnuts (raw)
- Water chestnuts

DAIRY

Dairy is an ideal Lung food because it provides so much lubrication for the Lungs. However, it is an example of what can happen when you get too much of a good thing. Too much dairy can cause congestion and produce dampness in the Lungs. If this is or has been a problem for you, substitute products made from cow's milk with products made from sheep's or goat's milk. All dairy products are good for the Lungs, including:

- Cheese (cow, goat, sheep, soy)
- Milk, whole and reduced fat (cow, goat, sheep, soy)
- Yogurt (cow, goat, sheep, soy)

OILS/BUTTER

The same caveat for dairy applies to butter. When cooking with fat choose from:

- Butter
- Olive oil
- Peanut oil
- Vegetable oil

BEVERAGES

Stay away from caffeinated soft drinks, tea, and coffee because they work like diuretics and will cause dryness in the Lungs. Mint, especially in hot weather, is good for the Lungs because it helps open the surface of the skin to let out heat and cool you down. Drink these teas iced or cold.

- Peppermint tea
- Spearmint tea

CONDIMENTS AND SPICES

Though hot and highly spiced cuisines are not for you, it does not mean that you must avoid all spices. Just minimize herbs and spices that add heat to food, and go light on the salt shaker. Good news: Sea salt is a Lung type's friend because of its ability to absorb water. However, if your doctor has you on a low-salt diet, do not start using salt without consulting with your doctor first. Lung-friendly condiments and spices include:

- Basil
- Bay leaf
- Cinnamon
- Coriander
- Garlic
- Ginger
- Honey
- Licorice
- Maltose
- Mint
- Mustard and mustard seeds
- Nutmeg
- Rosemary
- Royal jelly (liquid)
- Sea salt
- Sugar (cane)
- Wine for cooking

The Three-Day Lung Diet

This is a sample of what a typical Lung diet looks like. If you have any of the skin problems or illnesses described in this chapter, take advantage of dishes such as these to get you back on track to good Lung health. If you like to snack, opt for healthy foods, such as a handful of nuts or a piece of fruit from the list or a low-fat yogurt.

DAY 1

BREAKFAST

Scoop of cottage cheese
Rye toast with butter
Sliced peaches

LUNCH

Steamed Mussels with Shallots and Wine (page 132)
Spinach salad with sliced strawberries and toasted almonds
Whole wheat bread

DINNER

Roast Turkey Breast (page 135)
Baked Cauliflower with Béchamel Sauce (page 134)
Watercress or green salad with *Olive Oil and Lemon Dressing (page 137)*

DAY 2

BREAKFAST

Grapefruit
Whitefish salad on rye toast

LUNCH

Carrot Soup (page 136)
Baked Tofu and Eggplant (page 133)

DINNER

Roast duck breast
Baked yam
Steamed green beans

DAY 3

BREAKFAST

Whole grain cereal with milk with a sliced banana

Low-fat or nonfat yogurt

LUNCH

Grilled rosemary chicken

Steamed asparagus

Rice

Fruit cup

DINNER

Baked Tilapia (page 133)

Baked white potato

Steamed zucchini

Poached Pears (page 137)

Rejuvenating Recipes

These recipes are designed with emphasis on white foods and other foods that are Lung-friendly.

STEAMED MUSSELS WITH SHALLOTS AND WINE

A generous sprinkling of parsley adds color to this traditional Belgian standard.

2 tablespoons extra virgin olive oil

¼ cup minced shallots

¾ cup dry white wine

½ teaspoon sea salt

3 pounds mussels, cleaned

½ cup chopped fresh parsley

Freshly ground black pepper

Heat the oil in a medium stockpot over medium heat. Add the shallots and sauté until translucent, about 3 minutes.

2 Pour the wine into the pot, add the salt, then add the mussels. Raise the heat, cover, and steam the mussels until they open, stirring occasionally to move them around, about 5 minutes.

3 Divide the mussels and their cooking liquid among 4 bowls. Sprinkle with parsley and grind black pepper over the top.

SERVES 4

▦ BAKED TILAPIA

You can substitute any flaky white fish, such as flounder, for the tilapia.

4 tilapia fillets
½ tablespoon unsalted butter, melted
3 tablespoons lemon juice
I garlic clove, minced
I teaspoon dried parsley
Sea salt and freshly ground black pepper

1 Preheat the oven to 375°F.

2 Rinse the tilapia under cool water and pat dry with paper towels. Spray a baking dish large enough to hold the fish in a single layer with nonstick cooking spray and add the fillets. Drizzle with the butter and lemon juice and sprinkle with the garlic and parsley. Season with salt and pepper.

3 Bake until the fish is white and pulls apart with a fork, about 30 minutes.

SERVES 4

▦ BAKED TOFU AND EGGPLANT

East meets West in this vegetarian main meal. Eggplant is loaded with moisture.

⅓ cup soy sauce
2 tablespoons oyster sauce
2 tablespoons sugar
3 tablespoons vegetable oil, plus more if needed

1 16-ounce package firm tofu, cut into 2-inch chunks
1 large eggplant, peeled and cut into 1-by-3-inch strips
2 garlic cloves, minced
¼ cup chopped fresh basil

1 Combine the soy sauce, oyster sauce, and sugar in a small bowl and set aside.

2 Heat the oil over medium-high heat in a medium sauté pan. Add the tofu and brown it on all sides. Do not stir while browning. Remove it from the pan with tongs to a plate and set aside.

3 If needed, add more oil to the pan and heat it over medium-high heat. Add the eggplant and sauté for about 5 minutes. Add the garlic and sauté for 5 minutes more, until the eggplant can be easily pierced with a fork and is brown on all sides.

4 Return the tofu to the pan and add the soy sauce mixture. Stir gently until heated through. Sprinkle with the basil.

SERVES 4

BAKED CAULIFLOWER WITH BÉCHAMEL SAUCE

Yes, the classic white sauce known as béchamel is Lung-friendly, but it generally doesn't make it onto the list of healthy foods because it is so high in fat. This recipe cuts the fat by more than half.

For the cauliflower
1 large head cauliflower, leaves removed
1 tablespoon sea salt, plus more to season
2 tablespoons unsalted butter
Freshly ground black pepper
2 tablespoons freshly grated Parmesan cheese

For the sauce
4 tablespoons unsalted butter
2 tablespoons all-purpose flour
2 cups skim milk, warmed
Pinch ground nutmeg

Sea salt and freshly ground black pepper
2 tablespoons freshly grated Parmesan cheese
1 tablespoon low-fat farmer cheese

1   Prepare the cauliflower: Make a deep X-shaped cut in the stalk of the cauliflower with a sharp paring knife. Put the cauliflower in a pot just large enough to hold it and add water to cover. Add the salt. Bring to a boil and cook on medium-high until just tender enough so you can penetrate the head with a fork. Drain and set aside to cool. When cool enough to handle, break the head into florets.

2   Meanwhile, preheat the oven to 375°F and make the sauce: Melt the butter over medium-low heat in a small saucepan. Add the flour and stir until smooth, about 1 minute. Add the milk in a steady stream and stir until smooth. Add the nutmeg and season with salt and pepper. Bring to a low boil, remove from the heat, and add the Parmesan and farmer cheeses. Stir until the cheeses melt and blend.

3   Melt the butter for the cauliflower in a large sauté pan. Add the florets and season with salt and pepper. Cook until the cauliflower is soft, about 10 minutes.

4   Transfer the cauliflower to a heatproof baking dish and dust with the Parmesan cheese. Bake until the sauce bubbles and the top is browned, about 10 minutes.

SERVES 4

ROAST TURKEY BREAST

If you're a Lung type, a simple roasted turkey breast is a great way to get moistening food into your system.

1 5- to 6-pound bone-in turkey breast
1 lemon, cut into quarters
2 tablespoons unsalted butter, softened
Sea salt and freshly ground black pepper
1 tablespoon garlic powder
1 tablespoon paprika

1 Preheat the oven to 325°F.

2 Rinse the turkey breast in cold water and pat dry. Rub the turkey all over with the lemon quarters, one at a time. Let sit for 15 minutes.

3 Rub the turkey breast all over, including the cavity, with the softened butter. Season with salt and pepper. Set the turkey breast on a rack in a roasting pan and sprinkle with the garlic powder and paprika. Pour ¼ cup water into the bottom of the pan. Roast uncovered, basting every 20 minutes, until the interior registers 160°F, about 15 minutes per pound.

4 Remove from the oven and tent loosely with aluminum foil for 30 minutes before slicing.

SERVES 10 TO 12

▦ CARROT SOUP

This soup can be served hot or chilled.

1½ teaspoons sesame oil
10 large spring onions or scallions, sliced
1 pound carrots, peeled and coarsely chopped
1 large sweet potato, peeled and roughly chopped
2 14.5-ounce cans vegetable broth
1½ cups water
1 1-inch piece fresh ginger, peeled
1 teaspoon sea salt
Freshly ground white pepper
Snipped fresh chives for garnish

1 Heat the oil in a medium saucepan over medium-high heat. Add spring onions and cook until softened, stirring often, about 3 minutes.

2 Add the carrots, sweet potato, broth, and water and bring to a boil. Reduce the heat, cover, and simmer until the vegetables are soft, about 25 minutes. Strain the broth from the solids, reserving the broth.

3 Put the solids, ginger, salt, and pepper to taste in a food processor or blender and puree until smooth. Add 1 cup of reserved broth and puree about

1 minute more. Adjust the seasoning and amount of broth as desired. Garnish with chives before serving.

SERVES 4

▨ OLIVE OIL AND LEMON DRESSING

This is a simple dressing you can mix in a flash. I prefer it over bottled dressings because it's fresh-tasting and I know exactly what I'm getting.

2 tablespoons extra virgin olive oil
2 tablespoons fresh lemon juice
¼ teaspoon sea salt
¼ teaspoon freshly ground black pepper
¼ teaspoon garlic powder

Combine all the ingredients in a small jar with a tight-fitting lid. Shake well.

SERVES 1

▨ POACHED PEARS

4 pears, preferably Bosc
1 cup red wine
¾ cup honey
2 tablespoons fresh lemon juice
2 tablespoons ground cinnamon
2 tablespoons vanilla extract
4 tablespoons vanilla yogurt, whisked
4 spearmint leaves with stems

1 Peel and carefully core the pears, leaving the stem.

2 Combine the wine, honey, lemon juice, cinnamon, and vanilla in a medium pot and bring to a boil. Add the pears, reduce the heat, and simmer for 10 to 12 minutes. Turn the pears and continue to simmer for an additional 8 to 10 minutes, until they are tender. Remove the pears and let them cool.

3 Bring the wine sauce back to a boil over medium-high heat and boil until it is reduced by half.

4 Place each pear upright in an individual serving bowl. Pour the sauce over the pears. Garnish with a dollop of yogurt and a spearmint leaf.

SERVES 4

9-1-1 HEALING THERAPY: SUNBURN

Not only is sunburn painful, it also affects your Lung Qi and dries out your skin. When your skin gets overexposed to the sun, take remedial action fast with this soothing lubricant. It is cooling and will remove the heat.

Put 2 tablespoons of plain whole-milk yogurt in a small dish. Break open over the yogurt 1 capsule each of vitamin A, vitamin E, and aloe vera. Blend the nutrients into the yogurt and rub it into the sunburned area.

If the burn is particularly painful and red, peel and slice a white potato and place the slices over the affected area. Secure them with a piece of gauze and leave in place for 20 minutes. This remedy pulls out the heat and will help prevent blistering.

CARING FOR YOUR SKIN THE NATURAL WAY

Cleansing the face properly both day and night and using an exfoliant once a week are key to preventing your skin from becoming too dry or too oily. Face washes remove surface debris and maintain the cleanliness of your skin. Exfoliants remove dead debris at the cellular level. Exfoliating is important to your skin because removing dead debris allows your skin to breathe better. It also helps other beauty products you use to penetrate more deeply.

Chapter 11 offers daily rituals for maintaining normal, healthy skin. The following recipes are especially formulated for skin problems brought on by diminished flow of Lung Qi. When cleansing, use sour cream or whole-milk yogurt for dry skin and use kefir or low-fat yogurt if your skin is oily. Using these formulas, wash your face in the evening before bed and after you wake in the morning. Increase or decrease the ingredient proportions to suit your desired consistency or result. Before using any product, whether homemade or purchased, I recommend performing a skin allergy patch test (page 219).

⊞ SOUR CREAM SKIN CLEANSER FOR DRY SKIN

Rose essential oil helps increase moisture in the skin. The fat in the sour cream helps lubricate the skin, so make sure to use a whole-milk variety. This is an ideal and inexpensive cleanser for those plagued with dry skin. It is easy to mix, so make it fresh every time you use it.

2 tablespoons sour cream
1 drop rose essential oil

Put the sour cream in a small dish and add the essential oil with an eyedropper. Mix and massage it all over your face, being careful to avoid the eyes. Leave it on for 2 minutes. Rinse it off with warm water, using your hands or a soft washcloth.

⊞ KEFIR CLEANSER FOR OILY SKIN

Kefir curds, which look like small clumps of cauliflower, were first used in the Caucasus Mountains near the Eurasian region of Georgia. When combined with milk and fermented, live bacteria and yeast in kefir are excellent digestive enzymes for your intestines. When applied to your face, the lactic acid, naturally found in milk, and the live kefir critters suck the bacteria from your pimples, chomp on dead surface cells, and wash them down with your excess face oil. It sounds extraterrestrial, but the amazing result of baby-soft, clean skin is worth it. Kefir can be found in Trader Joe's and most health food stores. If you can't find kefir, use low-fat plain yogurt. This cleanser tends to be strong smelling, but the essential oil will mask the odor.

2 tablespoons unflavored kefir
1 drop eucalyptus essential oil

Put the kefir in a small bowl and add the eucalyptus essential oil with an eyedropper. Mix and massage it all over your face, being careful to avoid the eyes.

Leave it on for 2 minutes. Rinse it off with warm water, using your hands or a soft washcloth.

▦ VINEGAR AND LEMON TONER

A toner is a must for skin care. The skin has an acid mantle that protects it from harmful bacteria, which can invade pores and cause skin breakouts. For the Lung type with oily or acne-prone skin, this can be particularly problematic.

9 ounces cider vinegar
½ teaspoon freshly squeezed lemon juice
I ounce purified water

Combine the ingredients in a bowl and apply to your clean face with a piece of cotton. Rinse with cool water and apply your favorite moisturizer.

▦ BROWN SUGAR, YOGURT, AND FLAXSEED EXFOLIANT

Brown sugar and the natural lactic acid enzymes found in yogurt are great for removing dead surface skin cells. Flaxseed adds oil to your skin and replenishes lost moisture. The antimicrobial properties of honey help prevent breakouts.

2 tablespoons plain yogurt
2 teaspoons ground flaxseed
½ teaspoon brown sugar
I teaspoon honey

Combine all the ingredients in a bowl. Apply a thin layer of the mixture to your face and massage it into your skin for 20 seconds with upward circular strokes. Rinse with warm water and apply your favorite moisturizer.

⊞ STRAWBERRIES-AND-CREAM BLEMISH MASK

This mask will help resolve blemishes. Strawberries contain salicylic acid, which is the key ingredient in many over-the-counter and prescription acne skin care products.

> ½ cup hulled fresh strawberries
> 1 tablespoon sour cream
> 2 teaspoons honey

Combine the ingredients in a blender and blend until the mixture reaches a smooth and thick consistency. Apply in the evening on your face and neck, being careful to avoid the eye areas. Relax and let the mask sit for 15 minutes. Rinse with cool water, pat your skin dry, and apply your favorite moisturizer.

IF YOU DON'T WANT TO MAKE IT, THEN BUY IT . . .

Naturopathica Chamomile Cleansing Milk

Cost: About $28

Size: 5 oz.

A great basic cleanser and makeup remover for normal to dry skin. It combines the soothing, anti-inflammatory properties of German chamomile, the cleansing and purifying benefits of the moringa tree, and rose water for a gentle and effective cleansing milk.

Neal's Yard Remedies Palmarosa Facial Wash

Cost: About $22

Size: 100 ml

It's difficult to find a cleanser for oily skin that cleans your pores without drying the rest of your face, but this one does. This mild foaming wash for oily skin uses the oil extracted from palmarosa grass to gently clean oily areas and hydrate the rest.

The Organic Pharmacy Carrot Butter Cleanser

Cost: About $50

Size: 70 ml

The antioxidant property of carrots is blended with skin-softening shea and cocoa butter to dissolve dirt and grime. This cleanser also contains chamomile, rosemary, and lavender essential oils to soothe and decongest the skin. It is rich and creamy and perfect for very dry and irritated skin.

Yon-Ka Paris Lotion PS (normal to dry skin) or Lotion PG (normal to oily skin)
Cost: About $36

While Yon-Ka is still in the process of eliminating preservatives and parabens from its products, I had to mention these because you just can't beat them. The signature essential Yon-Ka five—lavender, geranium, rosemary, thyme, and cypress—are the perfect balance of fragrance and effectiveness. These after-cleansing face toners smell and feel so good you might be tempted to drink them.

Luzern Micro-Exfoliant Deep Hydrating Scrub
Cost: About $38
Size: 5 oz.

This ultra-gentle scrub uses fine jojoba beads, grapefruit, lemon, and cucumber to naturally exfoliate dead surface skin cells without irritating or scratching your skin. It decongests and refines clogged pores, smooths skin, and hydrates it. It makes your skin look and feel smooth and silky.

Naturopathica Moss Blemish Treatment

Cost: About $38

Size: .5 oz.

An effective spot treatment for blemishes, this lotion combines purifying extracts of moss to clean infected pores and reduce redness, bentonite clay to dry excess oil, and sulfur to help eliminate blackheads. It also removes excess oil, dries oily blemishes, and promotes clear skin.

8

Hot and Bothered: Calming the Heart

SEVERAL MONTHS AGO, LINDA, AGE FIFTY, CAME into my office visibly flustered and anxious. Her body, although soft and willowy, appeared edgy and tense as she nervously introduced herself. Her speech was quick and agitated. I immediately noted that her face was slightly red, her cheeks were flushed and irritated, and that she had small broken capillaries on her forehead, cheeks, and chin. I calmly ushered her into a treatment room and began her interview.

"I can't believe my complexion," she explained. "My skin used to be so rosy and soft. Now it's a mess, and no matter what I do I can't seem to get it under control. I have a drawer full of creams and products, and nothing works. I was browsing the Internet for advice and came across your website. So here I am."

Upon examination I noticed that she had patches of eczema on her elbows, and her hands were swollen and hot to the touch. I asked her if she frequently felt thirsty. She said, "I do drink a lot more water than I used to, but I attributed it to my changing hormones and my recent development of night sweats. Can you help me with that, too?"

"It's likely they're all related," I told her, "so, yes, acupuncture can help. But first I need to know a little bit more about you."

I asked her about other aspects of her life, including her sleep habits, moods, and emotions. She confided she was having some personal problems and could see that they were having a negative effect on her. Not only had she recently quit her job, but her marriage of twenty-five years was on the rocks. As a result, she said she felt anxious all the time and she was having difficulty falling asleep at night. When she finally did get to sleep, "scary dreams" woke her up.

"My moods are all over the place," she said. "I barely recognize myself. I used to be a social, friendly person. I used to love spending time with friends, going out at night, and entertaining guests at home. Now I can't remember the last time I enjoyed being with anyone. I constantly feel exhausted and agitated. I think about seeing someone for prescription medication for my anxiety and moodiness, but I'm reluctant to take drugs."

I could see that Linda was having problems of the Heart more complex than just her failing marriage.

Portrait of a Heart Type

Physically, a Heart type is sleek and willowy with a long neck and limbs, soft, smooth skin, and a rosy, glowing complexion. Heart types are warm and outgoing and love to talk and socialize. They are charismatic, generous, affectionate, expressive, and intuitive.

The Heart's orifice is the tongue, which means your ability to communicate clearly is related to your Heart. Because of this, Heart types are typically great communicators. Heart types make exemplary leaders, as they excel at empowering and motivating others into action. They are articulate and magnetic entertainers and thrive when they are the center of attention.

When the Heart is out of balance, it shows in the skin and complexion. The face can become pale and puffy with fine lines, or it can get red, flushed, irritated, and prone to broken capillaries—no surprise, since its element is fire. Heart types are susceptible to poor circulation, high or low blood pressure, heart palpitations, fatigue, and disturbed sleep. They also have a tendency to get mouth sores.

When the Heart is weak or overburdened, Heart types can lose their zest for life and compassion and become confused and demanding. Or they can become anxious or hyperactive, talk too fast and too much, stutter, or laugh nervously. Like Linda, a classic Heart type, people with an imbalance of Heart Qi suffer from anxiety, restlessness, and insomnia, and can have dream-disturbed sleep. Also like Linda, an imbalance in your Heart can be caused by emotional trauma, chronic stress, grief, and worry.

The Emotional Heart

Of all the Organs, the Heart is the most emotionally fragile. This is because the Heart controls emotional regulation. For a Heart type, managing emotions is like riding a roller coaster. The highs can be breathtakingly high, the lows can be a swift plunge into the doldrums, and there are a lot of twists and turns in between.

The Heart is also in charge of the emotion of joy. When the Heart is healthy, Heart types are the life of the party. They are enthusiastic, and have a great sense of humor, an optimistic outlook on life, and a kind, generous spirit. Not enough joy (feeling depressed) or too much joy (winning the lottery) can impact anyone's Heart Qi, but Heart types are the most vulnerable. For a Heart type with unhealthy Qi, mood swings are common.

The Role of the Heart: A Healthy Complexion

Chinese and Western medicine view the heart differently. In Western medicine, the Heart is the Organ that drives the circulatory system, which is responsible for transporting oxygen in your blood from the lungs and heart into arteries and capillaries and throughout the body. Once the oxygen has been used, blood is then returned to the lungs and heart through the veins. When the heart doesn't get enough oxygen, it damages the heart muscle, a common problem. Heart disease is the leading cause of death in the United States, as well as other industrialized countries, including the United Kingdom and Canada.

Chinese medicine concurs that the Heart is responsible for the circulation of blood and the health of the blood vessels. Likewise, Chinese medicine recognizes that a weak Heart can lead to chest pains, palpitations, or even a fatal heart attack. However, Chinese medicine sees a disruption of Heart Qi, and not just a reduction in oxygen flow, as the major cause of Heart problems.

Chinese medical doctrine also says your facial health—that is, the quality of your complexion—is related to the health of your Heart. This is because the Heart is responsible for nourishing the skin by maintaining proper flow of Blood. Your Heart is in charge of the integrity of your capillaries and your Blood circulation. When Heart Qi isn't flowing properly, it shows up on your face as either paleness with fine lines or a purplish-red complexion with broken capillaries, a condition known in Western medicine as telangiectasia. It is characterized by tiny twisted, red, bruiselike capillaries, frequently referred to as spider veins. They are most prominent on the cheeks, chin, nose, and forehead and are sometimes accompanied by red, itchy patches of dry skin.

Stereotypically, telangiectasia is associated with hard-core or frequent drinking, but anyone can develop it. Western medicine believes that, although the cause is unknown, it can be attributed to aging or possibly genetics. The condition is aggravated by washing your face with water that is too hot, scrubbing your face too hard, excessive exposure to the sun, eating spicy food, smoking or chewing tobacco, and drinking alcohol. Once broken, say Western doctors, these tiny spider veins or red blotchy patches cannot easily be reversed. Conventional treatments range from laser therapy to cosmetic surgery.

Eastern medicine recognizes this condition the same as Western doctors, but parts ways with Western medicine when it comes to cause and cure. While Eastern medicine agrees that the same factors aggravate the condition, it points to the underlying cause as an imbalance in your Heart Qi. Eastern medicine also believes that by correcting this problem—that is, by balancing your Heart Qi—you can minimize the symptoms without laser or surgical intervention. Acupuncture is an effective treatment.

Thinking and Acting with the Heart

Chinese medicine dictates that the Heart is the House of the Mind. It is your Heart, rather than your brain, that controls your mental activities. Although it can be a confusing concept to understand, the health of the Heart has a lot to do with behavior—the way you express yourself physically and verbally—which is why the tongue is the Heart's complementary orifice. The Heart also governs your ability to think and act clearly during the day and sleep soundly at night.

Chinese medicine sees the Heart as the King of Emotions. Although each Organ has its own emotional property, the Heart is unique because it controls your psyche, what Eastern medicine refers to as Shen. In Eastern medicine, how you behave and what you say is based on the way you perceive your immediate world. Psychological illness, known as a Shen disturbance, is perceived as a problem of the Heart rather than one of the brain. Mental illness and psychiatric disorders are addressed by treating the Heart.

How does this relate to your face? There is a common expression about the lovelorn that says some people wear their heart—their emotions—on their sleeve. In Chinese medicine, you wear your Heart—your thoughts, feelings, and emotions—on your face. The phrase "reading one's face" is a way of saying *I know what you are thinking from the expression on your face.*

As infants, we learn to communicate with the facial expressions that we send and receive. When we are happy, we smile. When discontent, we frown. We furrow our brows when we're confused and lift them when we "get it." We cry. We laugh. We wrinkle our nose. We flirt with our eyes, and we close them when we are sleepy or deep in thought.

The stressors in Linda's life, whether good (quitting her job) or bad (her failing marriage), were too much for her Heart to bear. Her sleep and erratic behavior were symptoms of the imbalance in her Heart. After twelve weeks of acupuncture to calm Linda's Shen, balance her Heart Qi, and cool her Heart Blood, plus a change in her home skin care regimen, Linda once again looked and felt like her radiant, glowing self. But there is more to her happy ending. Linda credits getting her Heart Qi flowing properly for a shift in her attitude that helped save her marriage. She also reconnected with her friends and social network, and once again she was able to sleep peacefully at night.

How the Heart Functions: Moving Blood and Qi

The Heart receives nutrients from the food and beverages you ingest by way of the Spleen and turns them into Blood. It then takes Qi from your Lungs and sends both Blood and Qi flowing in tandem to your face, Organs, and throughout your body. Because Qi moves Blood and Blood nourishes the Organs and regulates Qi, a deficiency of one affects the other. If your Heart Blood is weak, it will not be strong enough to move Qi. When this happens, it affects your complexion and health. Your face looks pale and puffy, you get fine lines all over, and you feel tired and sluggish, as if you were anemic.

When Qi and Blood can't move, they get stuck in your capillaries, which causes them to heat and swell. When the pressure becomes too great, fragile capillary walls break, a condition Eastern medicine calls Heat in the Blood. The result, as in Linda's case, is broken capillaries on the cheeks and a red flushed face. It also explains the eczema on her elbows, her swollen hands, her thirst, and her hot flashes. Linda was "on fire."

Your Heart's paired Organ is the Small Intestine. Similar to Western medicine, the Small Intestine receives digested food from the Stomach, and further sorts it into "clean" nutrients, which go to the Large Intestine for

---

FUNCTIONS OF THE HEART

The Heart teams up with the Small Intestine to perform these key functions:

- Transform food and energy into Blood
- Distribute Blood throughout the body
- Maintain the integrity of Blood vessels
- Create a healthy, radiant complexion
- Control emotions, thoughts, and actions

reabsorption, and "dirty" waste, which goes to the Bladder for excretion as urine. However, from a Chinese medicine point of view, the Small Intestine also filters mental "good" from "bad." The Small Intestine helps the Heart assess the difference between appropriate and inappropriate behavior. When Linda's Heart could no longer take the emotional extreme she was experiencing, her ability to rationally filter her emotions went on the blink.

Heart Guard: The Pericardium

Perhaps because the Heart is so precious and fragile, it is the only Organ of the five Organ systems that is linked to a sixth Organ system, the Pericardium, and its paired Organ, Triple Heater.

Just as it does in modern Western medicine, the Pericardium's job is to cover and protect the Heart from damage. Basically, it functions just like the Heart to control the flow of Blood, stabilize emotions, and influence thoughts. For the purposes of this book, the points on the Pericardium and Heart Meridians can be used interchangeably. The Pericardium and Triple Heater points used here target the cosmetic features associated with the Heart.

Unlike the other Organ systems, there is no corollary organ called Triple Heater. The role of the Triple Heater is controversial, even in Chinese medicine. Modern Chinese medicine experts postulate that the Triple Heater's role is to influence the flow of water through your body's connective tissue. Connective tissue supports all your body structures—your bones, muscles, organs, and so on. Like its name implies, connective tissue holds everything in place. In essence, it is the glue that keeps the body together.

Experts in classic Chinese medicine believe the role of the Triple Heater is to regulate the way water flows in and out of your Organs. Your body is divided into three sections, or "heaters"—upper, middle, and lower. The upper heater extends from your head to your chest and includes your Lungs and Heart. The middle heater extends from below your chest to your navel and contains your Spleen and Stomach. The lower heater is everything below your navel and is made up of the Liver, Kidneys, Bladder, and Small and Large Intestines. According to this theory, the Triple Heater acts as a superhighway that drops off water at each heater and takes away waste and debris.

By whatever method the Triple Heater functions, both modern and classical experts concur that massaging points on its pathway reduces puffiness and swelling, calms irritation, and cleanses your face and body.

The Heart's Evil: Beware of Fire

Heat is your body's fuel. You cannot function without it. Not only do you need heat to move around, you need heat to sit and read a book, and even understand the words on the page. You need heat to breathe, digest your food, and use what you've metabolized to make more heat. Too little or too much heat can cause Heart problems.

The Heart needs heat to do its job, and without enough heat the Heart loses its ability to circulate Blood. On the other hand, too much heat in the Heart causes it to catch on fire. Since fire usually rises, when you get "heat in the Heart," it affects your head and your brain. It causes capillaries to break on your face, your cheeks get flushed, dry, and irritated, and you sweat profusely. When Heart fire rises, it can wreak mental havoc, causing insomnia, agitation, and confusion.

CHARACTERISTICS OF A HEART TYPE

Signs of a Healthy Heart

- Rosy, glowing complexion
- Soft, smooth skin
- Sleek, willowy physique
- Healthy Blood circulation
- Restful sleep
- Ability to communicate clearly
- Appropriate thoughts and proper behavior

Signs of an Unhealthy Heart

- Pale, purplish, or red complexion
- Fine lines
- Flushed face
- Broken capillaries
- Sweating
- Poor Blood circulation
- Swollen hands
- Excessive thirst
- Insomnia
- Emotional fragility

Self-Acupressure for Good Circulation in the Face

This is an excellent routine for Heart types to help keep up the integrity of their complexion and avoid the broken capillaries and redness to which they are so vulnerable. However, anyone interested in maintaining good circulation to the face should do this massage. It can be done as a stand-alone treatment or integrated in the AcuFacial® Acupressure Facelift protocol.

Massage each point three times on both sides of the body in a clockwise rotation for ten rotations before moving on to the next body part. Read the section "Touch and Go: Key Acupressure Points" on page 30 before beginning this routine.

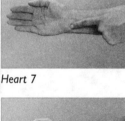

Heart 7

WRIST

Heart 7 | HT 7 is located on the inside wrist on the crease below the base of the hand. It is found on the spot between the tendons in line with the little finger. This is the primary point for balancing the Heart. It also relaxes the spirit.

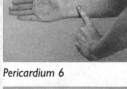

Pericardium 6

Pericardium 6 | P 6 is located on the inside of the lower arm, between the two tendons in the middle of the arm, three finger-widths from the crease of the wrist. Massaging this point balances Blood flow in the face by protecting and calming the Heart.

NECK

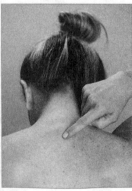

Governing Vessel 14

Governing Vessel 14 | If you slide your fingers from the top of your shoulder to the top of your spine you will find GV 14. It is located on top of the spine, between the seventh cervical and first thoracic vertebra. It strengthens the Heart Qi and can be used to lift and tone facial muscles, reduce facial puffiness, diminish sunspots, and brighten the face.

Triple Heater 17 | TH 17 is located in the depression below the ear at the base of the skull. In this routine, it clears heat and congestion from the face. Do both points at the same time, or one at a time, three times.

Small Intestine 17 | Slide your fingers forward to the long muscle extending from your jaw to your collarbone. This is SI 17. This point is used to open the neck and face.

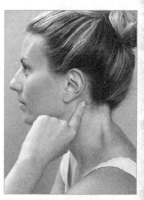

Triple Heater 17

FACE

Stomach 3 | This point is located directly below the center of your eye at the level of the nostrils. It opens and moves Qi and Blood in your cheeks and sinus area.

Stomach 7 | This point is located in front of your ear. You can find it by feeling for the depression between the cheekbone and the jawbone. It balances most of the nerves and vessels in your face.

Small Intestine 18 | This point is located on the cheek, directly below the outer edge of the eye and lateral to the side of the nose. It is used to tone Qi and Blood in the cheeks.

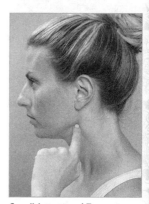

Small Intestine 17

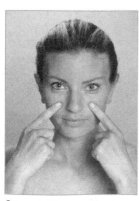

Stomach 3

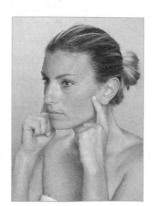

Stomach 7

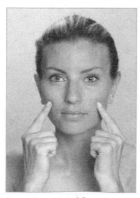

Small Intestine 18

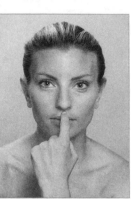

Governing Vessel 26

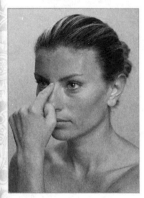

Yin Tang

Governing Vessel 26 | This point is located in the soft tissue below the tip of your nose and above the center of your upper lip. It increases circulation to the face and head and improves a pale or puffy complexion.

Yin Tang | This is an extra point located between the eyebrows. It clears the head and is extremely relaxing.

Diet for a Rosy Complexion

The Heart is most active—and most likely to act up—during the summer. This means that eating foods that deliver heat internally can create fire in the Heart. Cool Yin foods should dominate the diet of a Heart type, especially during the heat of the summer and for those who live in a warm climate.

COLOR ME RED

With the Heart's affinity to attract the evil fire, it's no wonder that its color is red! Unlike fire, however, red foods are good for the Heart. Make sure to include these foods in your diet.

- Apples
- Apricots
- Beets
- Bell peppers (red)
- Bitters
- Blood oranges
- Cabbage (red)
- Cherries
- Cinnamon
- Cranberries
- Grapefruit (pink and red)
- Grapes
- Guava
- Kidney beans
- Shrimp
- Strawberries
- Papaya
- Paprika
- Pears (red)
- Plums (red)
- Pomegranate
- Potatoes (red)
- Radicchio
- Radishes
- Raspberries (red)
- Red onions
- Rhubarb
- Tomatoes
- Watermelon

9-1-1 RESCUE REMEDY: BROKEN CAPILLARIES

Contrary to Western thinking, broken capillaries can be treated naturally and without drastic cosmetic therapy.

It is important to remember that broken capillaries as well as red, flushed skin should be treated tenderly. Wash your face gently with tepid water and a gentle milk-based cleanser. Wear a broad-spectrum sunblock every day, even in the winter. Sunblock not only protects you from sun damage but shields you from other harsh environmental elements as well. Eat the heat-clearing foods recommended in this chapter, particularly papaya, persimmons, adzuki and mung beans. Even more important, avoid alcohol, caffeine, fried foods, hot spices, and spicy foods, as they tend to aggravate internal heat.

In addition, use these points from the self-acupressure massage below until the redness fades, which could take weeks or months. Continue to do it two or three times a week to help prevent a recurrence. As with other routines, do each point in ten clockwise rotations before moving on to the next. Repeat the sequence three times. The instructions for these points can be found in the acupressure directions for the Heart.

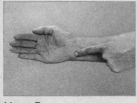

Heart 7

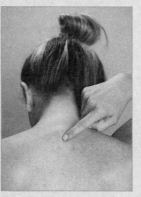

Governing Vessel 14

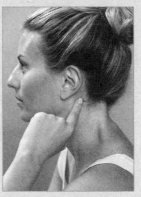

Triple Heater 17

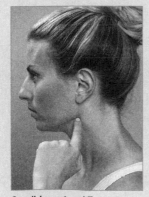

Small Intestine 17

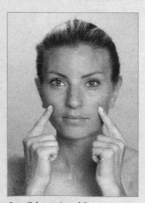

Small Intestine 18

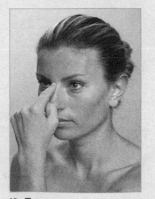

Yin Tang

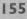

This also means avoiding hot spices and spicy foods, especially if and when you are hot Hearted. Cooling foods tend toward the green end of the spectrum—lettuce, cucumbers, and watercress are some of the coolest. Lean foods, such as most fish and seafood, are cooling, as are many vegetables. For the same reason, Heart types should avoid fried and greasy foods.

Heart types should be careful when eating meat, as most types are warming. Eat meat in moderation, and try to avoid eating it when the outside temperature is high. When you do eat meat, eat it in small portions, just a few ounces at a time. Eating meat in combination with vegetables, such as in a stew or as a kabob, is the best way to handle their heating effects.

Bitter is the preferred taste of Heart types. Bitter foods, such as kale, broccoli rabe, and chicory, help balance Heart Qi and Blood. So, too, does beer. Though coffee is a bitter flavor, it can aggravate Heart Qi when drunk in excess. Alcohol in all forms, including beer, should be enjoyed in moderation.

The following are the foods you should be targeting in your diet.

FISH, FOWL, MEAT

Even though the Heart's color is red, red meats should play a small role in your diet. You're best off leaning toward fish and seafood.

- Beef (lean)
- Chicken
- Clams
- Crab
- Egg yolks
- Lamb (in moderation)
- Oysters
- Shrimp

VEGETABLES

Vegetables dominate the Heart diet because they are cooling. Get as much of these vegetables, especially during the warm summer season.

- Asparagus
- Bamboo shoots
- Beets
- Bok choy
- Broccoli
- Broccoli rabe
- Cabbage
- Carrots
- Cauliflower
- Celery

- Chicory
- Chinese cabbage
- Corn
- Cucumber
- Dandelion greens
- Eggplant
- Kale
- Lettuce
- Mushrooms
- Onions
- Parsley
- Radishes
- Scallions
- Seaweed
- Snow peas
- Spinach
- Sprouts
- Summer squash
- Swiss chard
- Tomatoes
- Turnips
- Watercress
- Zucchini

FRUITS

These fruits are refreshing and cooling and complement a Heart diet.

- Apples
- Apricots
- Cantaloupe
- Lemons
- Mangos
- Oranges
- Papaya
- Peaches
- Pears
- Persimmons
- Plums
- Watermelon

GRAINS

Grains are great for balancing Organs. When choosing from the list below, whole grains are the best choice for the Heart.

- Barley
- Millet
- Rye
- Whole wheat flour

LEGUMES

Of all the legumes to choose from, adzuki and mung beans are the most cooling.

- Adzuki beans
- Mung beans
- Soybeans
- Tofu

NUTS AND SEEDS

Cardamom in its ground form appears in the spice aisle of almost any market, but cardamom seeds might be a little harder to find. Cardamom seeds, which are retrieved from pods, are indigenous to India; they can be found in specialty stores and Indian marketplaces. They are chewed whole and raw, and impart a refreshing taste.

- Cardamom seeds

OILS/BUTTER

When fat is called for in a recipe, opt for one of these. Safflower is the best, but the rest are acceptable.

- Butter
- Canola oil
- Olive oil
- Safflower oil
- Sesame oil

DAIRY

- Cheese (cow's milk)
- Milk (cow's)
- Yogurt (cow's milk)

BEVERAGES

These are the best cooling teas:

- Black tea (in moderation)
- Chrysanthemum tea
- Peppermint tea

CONDIMENTS AND SPICES

The Heart tends toward a "clean" diet, devoid of many spices. Favor these:

- Angostura bitters
- Brown sugar
- Cardamom
- Cilantro
- Dill
- Ginseng
- Honey
- Mint
- Mustard
- Vinegar (all varieties)

Three-Day Heart Menu

This is a sample of what a Heart diet looks like.

DAY 1

BREAKFAST

Cantaloupe
Low-fat cottage cheese
Rye toast
Mint tea

LUNCH

Crab and Asparagus Salad with Mustard Vinaigrette (page 165)
Plums

DINNER

Baked Red Snapper with Tomatoes and Lemon Broth (page 160)
Baked Beets (page 161)
Millet

DAY 2

BREAKFAST

Yogurt with mixed fruit
Rye toast
Tea

LUNCH
> *Gazpacho Garnished with Fresh Mint (page 162)*
> Clams steamed in beer

DINNER
> Roast chicken
> Sautéed bok choy
> *Summer Squash Salad (page 163)*
> *Red Raspberry Parfait (page 163)*

DAY 3

BREAKFAST
> Scrambled eggs
> Rye toast with apricot marmalade
> Herbal tea

LUNCH
> *Tofu and Vegetable Stir-Fry (page 164)* over whole wheat pasta
> *Tomatoes and Scallions (page 162)*

DINNER
> *Wok-Seared Shrimp with Snow Peas (page 164)*
> Pureed turnips
> Sliced tomato
> Poached pears
> Herb tea

BAKED RED SNAPPER WITH TOMATOES AND LEMON BROTH

The tomatoes and lemon broth give the fish a wonderful juiciness and fresh taste.

4 6- to 8-ounce red snapper fillets
1 teaspoon sea salt
Freshly ground black pepper
¼ cup fresh lemon juice
2 tablespoons extra virgin olive oil

1½ teaspoons minced garlic
1 teaspoon dried oregano
2 medium tomatoes, cored and cut crosswise into ¼-inch slices
1 tablespoon minced fresh parsley

1   Preheat the oven to 400°F and position a rack in the middle.

2   Wash the snapper fillets under cold water and dry with paper towels. Season them on both sides with the salt and a few grindings of black pepper.

3   Combine the lemon juice, oil, garlic, and ½ teaspoon of the oregano in a shallow baking just large enough to hold the fillets in one layer. Stir until well blended. Add the fillets and turn them a few times to coat them evenly with the mixture. Turn the fillets skin side down.

4   Place the tomato slices over the fillets and sprinkle with the remaining ½ teaspoon oregano. Bake for 10 to 12 minutes, until the fillets flake easily when pressed gently with a fork. Sprinkle with the parsley and serve immediately directly from the baking dish.

SERVES 4

BAKED BEETS

10 small fresh red beets
2 tablespoons unsalted butter, melted
1 tablespoon finely chopped onion
1 tablespoon lemon juice
1 teaspoon sea salt
⅛ teaspoon freshly ground black pepper

1   Preheat the oven to 400°F.

2   Peel the beets and slice them ¼-inch thick. Place the beets in a medium casserole dish sprayed with nonstick spray. Combine the remaining ingredients and pour the mixture over the beets. Cover and bake for 30 minutes or until they are easily pierced with a fork.

SERVES 4

▦ GAZPACHO GARNISHED WITH FRESH MINT

2 14-ounce cans diced tomatoes
½ cup water
2 tablespoons olive oil
½ cup crumbled feta cheese
1 cup diced seeded watermelon, cut into ¼-inch cubes
1 seedless cucumber, cut into ¼-inch slices
1 small red onion, diced into ¼-inch pieces
1 small yellow bell pepper, seeded and diced into ¼-inch pieces
1 small jalapeño, seeded and cut into ¼-inch pieces
2 tablespoons sherry vinegar
2 tablespoons chopped cilantro
4 sprigs fresh mint, for garnish
Sea salt and freshly ground black pepper

1 Process ½ cup of the tomatoes with the oil and water in a blender or food processor until pureed.

2 Pour the puree into a bowl large enough to accommodate all the ingredients, and add the remaining ingredients.

3 Mix and refrigerate. Serve cool.

SERVES 4

▦ TOMATOES AND SCALLIONS

2 large tomatoes, sliced
4 scallions, coarsely chopped
1 teaspoon dried oregano
Dash sea salt
2 tablespoons extra virgin olive oil

Arrange the tomato slices on a serving platter. Sprinkle with the scallions, oregano, and salt and drizzle with the oil. Let stand for 10 minutes before serving.

SERVES 4

▦ RED RASPBERRY PARFAIT

I cup red raspberries
Juice of ½ lemon
I cup thin apple slices, cut in half
I cup thin mango slices, cut in half
4 tablespoons honey
4 mint leaves

I   Wash and pat the raspberries dry. Squeeze the lemon over the apple slices.

2   Divide half of the raspberries among 4 parfait glasses. Alternate layers of apples and mangos, and end with the remaining raspberries. Drizzle I tablespoon of honey on top of each parfait and garnish with a mint leaf.

SERVES 4

▦ SUMMER SQUASH SALAD

3 medium summer (yellow) squash
2 medium zucchini
½ medium red onion, thinly sliced
2 tablespoons canola oil
Juice of I small lemon
Sea salt and freshly ground black pepper

I   Cut the squashes horizontally into ½-inch slices. Steam them in a vegetable steamer for 10 minutes, or until soft.

2   Put the squash in a medium bowl and mash lightly with a potato masher. Cool, then cover and refrigerate for 30 minutes. Drain any liquid that may have accumulated. Add the onion, oil, and lemon juice and season with salt and pepper. Serve cold as a side dish or salad.

SERVES 4

✦ WOK-SEARED SHRIMP WITH SNOW PEAS

Cooking with a wok is easy; your food is cooked quickly, meaning you aren't losing nutrients. This recipe and the next are best when prepared in a wok.

¼ cup water
1 tablespoon rice vinegar
⅛ teaspoon sesame oil
½ teaspoon cornstarch
¼ teaspoon sea salt
2 dashes freshly ground black pepper
2 teaspoons canola oil
5 slices fresh ginger
1½ pounds cooked shrimp, peeled
3 ounces snow peas

1 Combine the water, rice vinegar, and sesame oil in a small bowl. Stir in the cornstarch until dissolved. Add the salt and pepper.

2 Heat a wok over high heat and add the canola oil. Add the ginger and stir-fry until aromatic, about 30 seconds. Be careful not to burn the ginger.

3 Add the shrimp and toss in the wok a few times or stir well. Add snow peas and the reserved liquid. Toss to coat the shrimp. Cook approximately 2 minutes, until the shrimp are pink on the outside and opaque in the middle.

SERVES 4

✦ TOFU AND VEGETABLE STIR-FRY

1 tablespoon canola oil
½ medium onion, sliced
2 garlic cloves, minced
1 tablespoon diced ginger
1 16-ounce package tofu, drained and cut into ½-inch cubes
¾ cup haricots verts, cut in half
¾ cup peeled eggplant, cut into ¾-inch pieces
8 pencil-thin asparagus spears, trimmed and cut into ½-inch pieces

1 red bell pepper, cut into ½-inch strips
1 medium carrot, thinly sliced
1 small head bok choy, chopped
2 cups thinly sliced mushrooms
1¼ cups bean sprouts
1 cup bamboo shoots, drained and chopped
½ teaspoon crushed red pepper
½ cup water
¼ cup rice vinegar
2 tablespoons honey
2 tablespoons soy sauce
2 tablespoons cornstarch dissolved in 2 tablespoons water
2 medium scallions, thinly sliced on the diagonal into ½-inch pieces

1   Heat the oil in a large wok over medium-high heat. Add the onion and cook for 1 minute. Add the garlic and ginger and cook for 30 seconds. Add the tofu and cook approximately 1 minute, until golden brown.

2   Add the haricots verts, eggplant, asparagus, bell pepper, and carrot and cook for 2 minutes. Add the bok choy, mushrooms, bean sprouts, bamboo shoots, and crushed red pepper. Heat thoroughly, about 1 minute. Remove from the heat and set aside.

3   In a small saucepan, combine the water, vinegar, honey, and soy sauce and bring to a simmer. Cook for 2 minutes. Stir in the cornstarch and simmer until the sauce thickens. Pour it over the vegetables and tofu and garnish with the scallions.

SERVES 4

CRAB AND ASPARAGUS SALAD WITH MUSTARD VINAIGRETTE

A main dish salad—perfect for a spring or summer luncheon.

1 pound thin asparagus
1 head Bibb lettuce, torn into bite-size pieces
1 pound lump crabmeat, well drained
1 large tomato, diced

Vinaigrette
2 tablespoons balsamic vinegar
1 teaspoon Dijon mustard
1 garlic clove, smashed
1 shallot, diced
½ cup safflower or canola oil
Pinch of dried parsley
Sea salt and freshly ground black pepper

1 Trim the asparagus. Steam in a vegetable steamer until fork-tender, but not too soft, about 5 minutes. Set aside to cool.

2 Make the vinaigrette: In a small bowl, combine the vinegar, mustard, garlic, and shallot and mix well. Slowly whisk in the oil. Add the parsley and season with salt and pepper.

3 Divide the lettuce among 4 serving plates. Top with the crabmeat and tomato and drizzle with the dressing.

SERVES 4

Skin Care for a Healthy Complexion

For Heart types, the key to caring for the skin is to prevent heat and inflammation. The way to do so is to keep your face clean and cool with soothing creams. Using a skin cream daily, morning and night, is a must for a healthy complexion, especially if you're a Heart type. Apply it after cleansing your face and applying serum. Increase or decrease the ingredient proportions to suit your desired consistency or result. Before using any product, whether homemade or purchased, I recommend performing a skin allergy patch test (page 219).

SOOTHING FACE CREAM FOR RED, BLOTCHY SKIN

The oils and glycerin soothe the skin while chamomile and vitamin E ease the redness and irritation. Grapefruit extract and geranium help reduce inflammation and purify your skin. The vitamin E can be broken out of a capsule. This day cream can also be used at night.

> 2 tablespoons coconut oil (cooking oil)
> ⅓ cup evening primrose oil
> 1 tablespoon vegetable glycerin
> 1 teaspoon vitamin E, broken from a capsule
> ⅓ cup lukewarm chamomile tea
> 4 drops grapefruit seed extract
> 3 drops rose geranium essential oil

1 Stir together the coconut and primrose oils and the glycerin. Add the vitamin E and blend gently until smooth.

2 Slowly pour the tea into the oil, stirring constantly with a fork or wire whisk until the mixture is smooth. Stir in the grapefruit seed extract and rose geranium essential oil.

3 Pour the mixture into a clean, dark glass container with a tight-fitting lid. Allow it to cool before putting on the lid, stirring the mixture occasionally as it cools to prevent the ingredients from separating. Store in a cool, dark place and shake well before using.

SOOTHING FACE CREAM FOR DRY, IRRITATED SKIN

This is particularly good as a night cream because it's very rich. In addition to the difference it makes in your skin, the calming floral scents of the essential oils help soothe the mind and balance the Heart's emotions.

> 2 tablespoons coconut oil (cooking oil)
> ⅓ cup avocado oil
> 1 tablespoon vegetable glycerin
> 1 teaspoon vitamin E, broken from a capsule
> ⅓ cup rose water
> 10 drops grapefruit seed extract
> 4 drops sandalwood essential oil
> 3 drops patchouli essential oil

1 drop rosewood essential oil
1 drop rose geranium essential oil
1 drop ylang-ylang essential oil

1 Stir together the coconut and avocado oils and the glycerin. Add the vitamin E and gently blend until smooth.

2 Warm the rose water in a small pot to lukewarm. Slowly pour the warmed water into the oil, stirring constantly with a fork or wire whisk until the mixture is smooth. Add the grapefruit seed extract and essential oils.

3 Pour the mixture into a clean, dark 6-ounce glass jar. Allow the cream to cool before putting on the lid, stirring the mixture occasionally as it cools to prevent the ingredients from separating. Store in a cool, dark place.

SUN-FREE SUNBLOCK

This silky, water-resistant sunblock for the face comes from Australia, where the summers are hot and the sun is very strong. Although the sunblock is effective, Heart types (and others) should still beware of the sun!

½ cup coconut oil (cooking oil)
½ cup jojoba oil
¼ cup zinc oxide
2 tablespoons titanium oxide

1 Combine the coconut and jojoba oils in a bowl. Mix in the zinc oxide and titanium oxide.

2 Apply to your face liberally 20 minutes before sun exposure and repeat every 2 hours.

IF YOU DON'T WANT TO MAKE IT, THEN BUY IT . . .

Aubrey Organics Vegecol with Aloe Moisturizing Cream
Cost: About $15
Size: 4 oz.
This formula uses aloe vera and calendula to soothe and restore moisture to irritated skin. Horsetail and coltsfoot are added to tone skin and improve

elasticity. St. John's wort oil and coneflower oil help replenish moisture and smooth and firm skin.

Éminence Organic Skin Care of Hungary
Calm Skin Chamomile Moisture
Cost: About $58
Size: 2 oz.
This product soothes and moisturizes sensitive and rosacea-prone skin. Chamomile tea, calendula oil, shea butter, and aloe vera calm and balance irritated skin.

Éminence Organics of Hungary
Rosehip Whip Moisturizer
Cost: About $58
Size: 2 oz.
This light moisturizer for oily, reactive skin uses rosehips to soothe and tone the skin, lemon juice to refresh the skin, and carrot juice and pectin to nourish and gently moisturize without clogging pores.

If you have sensitive skin, you must use sunscreen or sunblock to protect your face from harmful and irritating sun rays. These are good choices:

Badger SPF 30 Sunscreen
Cost: About $16
Size: 2.9 oz.
Badger sunscreen is a completely chemical-free lotion that is water-resistant for up to forty minutes. It provides broad-spectrum protection against both UVA and UVB rays. It is safe to use on kids. The primary active ingredient is zinc oxide. Other skin-nourishing ingredients include extra virgin olive oil, beeswax, jojoba oil, cocoa butter, and shea butter.

Alba Botanica Natural Very Emollient Sunblock Facial
Cost: About $10
Size: 4 oz.
A light but still rich sunblock that protects and nourishes the skin with aloe, calendula, chamomile extract, and more.

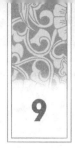

9

Wrinkles and Sunspots: Love the Liver

STUART, ATHLETICALLY BUILT WITH ROBUST muscles and thick, firm skin, was just shy of forty when he came to see me. He didn't like the way his handsome face was aging. He immediately started to complain about the wrinkles across his forehead and the fine lines surrounding his eyes. What really bothered him the most, however, was the deep crease between his eyebrows that was starting to give him a permanent scowl. He swore he wasn't vain and said he never dreamed he'd end up seeking cosmetic advice, but he was just too bothered by his appearance to ignore it.

"There are tons of guys who age well, and it's something that I really was never concerned about," he rambled as I took the pulse in both of his wrists. "Wrinkles are supposed to give you character, right? But not on me—I don't want them."

I smiled. "You're hardly alone. A lot of men feel the way you do and just accept it as a fact of life. That's not *exactly* the case. You don't have to have wrinkles—they are not just a fact of life."

I could tell from the enthusiastic way Stuart described his life that he loved his job on Wall Street and the fast-paced routine of his daily life—a typical New Yorker, stressed and always on the go. At the sound of the weekday five-thirty a.m. alarm, he could fly out of bed, shower, and be dressed to the nines in no time flat. "All I need is a cup of coffee and I'm out the door," he said matter-of-factly. "The morning alarm is no problem for me, no matter how late I'm up the night before." He even had time to stop and pick up another cup of joe and a bagel with butter before hitting his desk by seven. He had it all gulped down and was raring to go at the sound of the stock market bell at nine-thirty.

Lunch, on the days he even bothered, was also on the run, usually a deli sandwich—roast beef or meatball—and a diet soda, which he inhaled while on the computer or in a meeting. "Lately it's been giving me a lot of heartburn," he said, admonishing his on-the-go eating habits. After work it was rush, rush to the gym to exercise. Before heading home or out for a business dinner, Stuart liked to stop for a cocktail or two. It was his way of unwinding.

Stuart was a master multitasker and proud of it, and although he performed well under pressure, he admitted the magnitude of his job was starting to get to him. He often found himself in quiet fits of anger and confided he surprised himself recently when he lashed out at a colleague. He didn't like where it all might be heading, and it was making him feel stressed and frustrated.

What he didn't mention was the periodic twitch in his right eyelid I noticed as we talked about his current state of health. When I asked him about his brittle-looking nails, he shrugged it off and blamed it on the weather. However, he said he couldn't explain the bouts of headaches that seemed to be getting more frequent or his neck and shoulder pain. "Think I should see a chiropractor?" he asked.

"I think we can handle it," I said. "Let's see what a little acupuncture and a change in your diet will do."

I had Stuart pegged from the start. He was a classic Liver type. From the viewpoint of Eastern

> ### SNAPSHOT OF THE
> ### LIVER
>
> *Element:* Wood
> *Complementary organ:* Gallbladder
> *Primary function:* Controlling the flow of Qi
> *Facial concern:* Wrinkles
> *Complementary orifice:* Eyes
> *Season:* Spring
> *Emotional regulation:* Anger
> *Color:* Green
> *Taste:* Sour
> *Primary evil:* Wind
> *Active time:* 11 p.m. to 3 a.m.

healers, Stuart's Liver Qi was completely out of balance. "The reason you are bothered by your appearance is that it isn't the way your face would age if your Liver was balanced," I explained. "In order to soften your forehead muscles and wrinkles, I am going to treat your Liver and get your Qi flowing smoothly. Weekly acupuncture treatments will help a lot, but you also need to change your habits and diet, and that includes reducing your drinking."

Stuart agreed and was eager to start. He modified his diet, got more rest (on the weekends), and did acupressure in addition to the weekly acupuncture treatments. On his fifth visit he reported that his headaches and neck and shoulder pain were gone, and his eyelid was no longer twitching. On his sixth visit he was beaming. "People are starting to ask me if I'm getting Botox!" he said with a smile. "Life is good."

Profile of a Liver Type

Healthy Liver types have thick, firm skin and solid, robust muscle tone. They are competitive, confident, seek challenges, crave adventure, and love action. They are driven to come in first and be the best at what they do. They also make great leaders. They excel at planning and decision making, and they have clear visions and goals and know how to accomplish them.

Liver types are doers. They like to accomplish their goals *yesterday*. So when something or someone gets in the way, it impedes their Liver movement. A healthy Liver type has the fluidity to roll with the punches and even use them to their advantage. An unhealthy Liver type, however, feels stifled, restrained, and frustrated, and angers easily. For example, if you quickly grow irritable when stuck in traffic, feel like you can't get where you want to go fast enough, or develop a case of road rage, it's a sign that your Liver is out of balance. In fact, Liver types are more affected by a stressful lifestyle than any other Organ type. As you've learned in the preceding chapters, Kidney types become fearful, Spleen types worry, Lung types get sad, and Heart types become anxious. But Liver types get angry. Anger in Eastern medicine includes feelings of frustration, irritability, and resentment.

When the Liver is hindered, Liver types can lose all perspective when it comes to keeping life in balance. They can be workaholics, with or without a clear direction. Emotionally, they may have difficulty expressing their anger or have bouts of rage, especially when feeling stressed, frustrated, or irritated. They can also be intolerant, impatient, and impulsive. This is what happened to Stuart.

When the Liver gets out of balance, it shows up in looks, as well as actions. Liver types will develop exaggerated wrinkles between the eyebrows, across the forehead, and around the eyes. Like Stuart, they are prone to eye problems—eyelid twitches, itchy eyes, and blurred vision are part of the package of a Liver in distress. So, too, are headaches and muscle spasms. When left untreated, people with a Liver problem can develop painful sciatica or nerve pain. Liver types are also prone to digestive discomfort, and menstrual disorders can develop in women.

For Stuart, acupuncture was a giant step in reversing his Liver trouble, but his combination of symptoms—the deep wrinkles, his twitching eye, his constant headaches, and his change in attitude—also called for a change in diet. I recommended that he stop the morning bagel and instead breakfast on whole wheat toast with sesame butter and fresh fruit or jam. I suggested he eat more greens and forgo the deli sandwich for a spinach salad with chicken breast for lunch. I also told him to eat seafood and fish, cut down on the caffeine, and reduce his alcohol consumption. I showed him acupressure points to massage for his head, neck, and shoulder tension.

Within a short period of time Stuart looked and felt better. Even though his job responsibilities had not changed, he said his attitude about them had. He felt more relaxed and less stressed, and he noticed that situations that bothered him in the past no longer did. Stuart thought that his overall performance had improved, especially when his boss complimented him on his excellent handling of a difficult client.

The Role of the Liver: Wrinkle-Free Skin

Smooth, wrinkle-free skin? That's a sign of a healthy Liver. The Liver is responsible for the contraction of your muscles, and it governs the process that prevents skin from wrinkling by maintaining a harmonious flow of Qi in your face and throughout your body and Organs.

When your Liver Qi moves smoothly, your muscles contract and relax evenly and the muscle attachments—your skin, ligaments, and tendons— move fluidly as well. When you have a healthy Liver, your skin is wrinkle-free, soft, and smooth, because the muscles and skin on your face move back and forth evenly.

You see, the muscles of your face differ from those of the rest of your body. The muscles of your body attach from either bone to bone, or from bone to tendon or ligament. Contracting these muscles moves your bones. This is apparent when you "make a muscle." Contract your upper arm muscle and you'll see your lower arm bend as your upper and lower arm bones move closer together. This is because tightening the muscles of your upper arm pulls and lifts the bones of your lower arm. When you relax your upper arm muscle, your lower arm bones relax as well.

Facial muscles are unique because they attach on one end to a bone or a muscle and on the other end to a muscle or your skin. When contracting a face muscle, it is your muscles and skin, rather than your bones, that move. The cheek muscles attach on one end to your cheekbone and on the other end to the muscles surrounding the outer corner of your mouth. Look in the mirror and smile and you will see that by contracting these muscles you pull the corner of your mouth upward toward your ear. You may also notice that the skin covering your cheeks lifts, folds, and creases around these contracted muscles. When you stop smiling, your cheek muscles relax and your skin resumes its smooth, flat appearance.

When you concentrate or scowl, you contract the muscles of your forehead and those that surround and support your eyes. When this happens, your skin and eyebrows move closer together. The result is a creasing of skin between your eyebrows—what is commonly referred to as "furrowing your brows." Relax your eye and forehead muscles, and the creases between your brows, on your forehead, and around your eyes may disappear.

Imagine your face muscles as an accordion and your skin as a thin piece of paper attached from end to end and stretched tightly across the surface. When you press the ends of the accordion or contract your muscles, the paper, or your skin, has less surface area to cover, so it folds and creases. With continuous folding over time, the paper weakens, causing it to lose its integrity. The paper starts to show signs of wear and eventually the creases remain visible, even when the "accordion" is not contracting. Over time the creases start to remain visible on your face as well. That's the day when you start to notice that you've got wrinkles.

Both Western medicine and Eastern medicine agree that wrinkles are formed by this kind of repetitive folding and constant contraction of facial muscles. Western medicine says it's inevitable and a natural part of the aging process—and that there's not a whole lot you can do about it short of Botox, dermabrasion, laser for skin tightening, or other topically invasive measures.

Likewise, Eastern medicine recognizes wrinkles as part of the aging process but believes anyone can delay, minimize, and even *prevent* wrinkling by keeping the Liver Qi even and free flowing. Healthy Liver Qi means muscles contract and relax with ease.

How the Liver Functions: An Abundance of Blood

The Liver has the essential job of distributing vital Blood to other Organs and throughout the body. The smooth and harmonious flow of Liver Blood is dependent upon Liver Qi. After your Heart collects Spleen essence, it turns it into Blood and sends it to the Liver, where it is stored. When you are active, you call on the Liver to release Blood, which joins Qi for passage through your Meridians and Organs to nourish and energize your body. When you are at rest, Blood returns to the Liver, where it remains until it is once again needed. If the Heart cannot produce enough Blood, or if the Liver fails to store or circulate it properly, it can affect more than your facial appearance. It impacts the health of your Organs and your entire body.

Just as a plant is dependent on water to survive, your muscles and body depend upon Liver Blood to thrive. When you do not have enough Blood, then muscle fibers, tendons, and ligaments lack the fluid needed to contract and relax smoothly. Movement through the Meridians and Organs slows down. Eventually Blood starts to congeal and Liver Qi rebels by separating itself from Blood. Void of Blood, Liver Qi begins to behave erratically. It can unpredictably fly upward instead of downward, downward instead of upward, speed up, slow down and, like a tornado, damage everything that is in its path.

The aftermath is muscles that move erratically and have difficulty relaxing, setting you up for the progressive formation of wrinkles on your face, among other problems. You might start to notice eye irritation, headaches, and neck and shoulder pain. Like Stuart, you could develop an eyelid twitch.

You can also develop muscle spasms, sciatica, or shooting pain throughout your body.

Other signs of poor Liver Blood flow are dry skin, brittle nails, headaches, dizziness, and weakness and numbness in your extremities. People with a sluggish Liver are susceptible to brown patches on the skin, which are commonly called sunspots. (Ironically, these brown patches were called liver spots until Western medicine decided they had nothing to do with a sick liver. However, in Chinese medicine, it has everything to do with your *Liver*.)

If your Liver Qi is out of balance for too long it can "flare." Similar to getting overheated, it makes you feel hot. Your face gets flushed, and your eyes get red and start to burn.

Also bearing the brunt of all this turmoil is the Liver's paired Organ, the Gallbladder. The Gallbladder's job is to store and secrete bile, which is essential to moving nourishment through the Stomach and Large Intestine. When the Liver is impaired, bile production slows, causing the digestive discomforts we know as heartburn and acid reflux.

The Liver's Evil: Wind

When the Liver gets weak, it is prone to the Eastern medicine evil known as wind. When the wind in the atmosphere begins to blow, it stirs and moves

---

FUNCTIONS OF THE LIVER

The Liver teams up with the Gallbladder to perform these key functions:

- Move Qi smoothly throughout the Organs and the entire body
- Store and regulate Blood volume
- Maintain even tendon, ligament, and muscle movement
- Maintain smooth skin and muscle contraction to prevent wrinkles
- Promote healthy nails
- Maintain healthy eyes and vision
- Protect against sunspots
- Help the body cope with stressful situations
- Control frustration and anger

everything in its path. Similarly, when wind blows internally, it stirs and agitates Liver Qi and Blood and has the capacity to create even greater chaos. The smooth and relaxed muscle movements that are the hallmark of a healthy Liver can cause irregular, disjointed, and spastic movements within itself and the entire body. Signs of wind agitating the Liver are facial tics, tremors, dizziness, and, in extreme cases, convulsions. Curiously, another sign of internal wind invasion is the lack of movement, or paralysis. Bell's palsy and facial paralysis are two examples of wind getting lodged in the muscles and channels, causing them to stiffen.

CHARACTERISTICS OF A LIVER TYPE

Signs of a healthy Liver are:

- Thick, firm skin
- Smooth, wrinkle-free face
- Strong, robust body and muscle tone
- Even muscle contraction
- Bright eyes and healthy vision
- Healthy nails
- An active and adventurous nature
- Calm, even-tempered disposition
- Clear mind and focused goals

Signs of an unhealthy Liver are:

- Wrinkles, particularly around the eyes and forehead
- Weak joints, tendons, and ligaments
- Muscle tension, especially in the neck and shoulders
- Sciatic pain
- Red, irritated eyes
- Vision problems, such as spasms, tics, and weak vision
- Sunspots
- Brittle nails
- Chronic heartburn
- Anger, frustration, and irritability
- Menstrual disorders

A Systemic Problem

Because the Liver is responsible for the smooth flow of Qi throughout the body and Organs, a constrained Liver can tax other Organs, particularly the Spleen and Lungs.

The Liver has a rather sensitive relationship with the Spleen. The Spleen craves stability, and the Liver likes movement. When the Liver cannot efficiently move Blood and Qi, it harms the Spleen, a condition Eastern medicine calls Liver invading the Spleen. When this happens, confusions reigns for Liver types. They can get caught in the middle of the two extremes. They may find themselves struggling with thoughts such as, *Should I say something or not? Do something or nothing? Move or stay still?* They also can experience signs of Spleen dampness, which manifests in another cosmetic problem akin to wrinkles: sagging facial muscles. This can affect your facial appearance even more by causing heaviness and sagging in the jowl area. It can also cause the same digestive problems experienced by Spleen types and, in women, cause irregularity in the menstrual cycle. (You can read more about Spleen dampness starting on page 88.)

When the Liver attacks the Lungs, it creates a dilemma between your ability to express (Liver) or repress (Lung). This creates mental conflict between expressing emotion and indifference, action and restraint, and chaos and order. Physically this can manifest as a breakout of pimples or acne, wheezing, tightness in the throat, or pain in the ribs.

Self-Acupressure to Soften Wrinkles

Liver types have a tendency to store a lot of tension in the face. The muscles of the brow and forehead get so tight that it's difficult to relax them. Not only does this contribute to wrinkles, it aggravates and can worsen already existing deep creases at the brow and on the forehead. This eight-point massage relaxes the muscles of the eyes and brow, which helps soften wrinkles in this area as well as prevent them.

This massage starts with the feet and works its way to the face. You'll do each massage on both sides of the body in a clockwise rotation for ten rotations. Do the entire routine three times before moving on to the next body part. Read the section "Touch and Go: Key Acupressure Points" on page 30 for instructions on how to do acupressure massage properly before beginning this routine.

FEET

Liver 2 | LV 2 is located on top of the foot at the base of the webbing between the big toe and second toe. In addition to smoothing wrinkles, it helps alleviate eyelid twitching and facial spasms.

Liver 3 | Slide your finger about one finger-width toward your ankle. This is LV 3. It helps soften wrinkles and clear Liver congestion.

Gallbladder 43 | Now, move to your little toe. GB 43 is located at the webbing between the little toe and fourth toe. This point helps soften wrinkles.

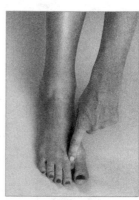
Liver 2

KNEE

Gallbladder 34 | Move up your legs to your knees. GB 34 is located on the outside of the knee on the indentation at the top of the large leg bone (fibula). This point helps resolve any issue associated with a Liver Qi imbalance.

HANDS

Large Intestine 4 | Hold your hand straight up and press your thumb to your index finger. LI 4 is located at the end of the crease between the two digits. This point addresses all imbalances in the face.

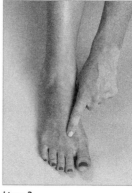
Liver 3

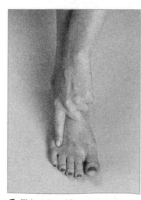
Gallbladder 43

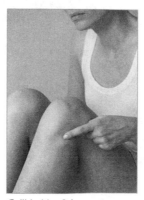
Gallbladder 34

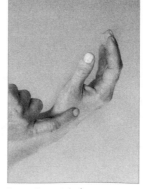
Large Intestine 4

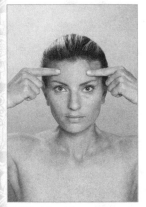

Gallbladder 20

HEAD

Gallbladder 20 | Place your index fingers in the center of your spine, below the base of your skull. Move your fingers toward your ears approximately two finger-widths to the indentation in front of the tendon. This is GB 20. In addition to relaxing muscle tension and easing wrinkles, this point opens Liver Qi to the head.

Gallbladder 14 | Bring your hands around to your forehead. GB 14 is located one finger-width above the center of the eyebrow. This point softens creases on the center and side of the forehead.

Gallbladder 14

9-1-1 RESCUE THERAPY: HEADACHES

Headaches come in several varieties, but if you are plagued by tension headaches or cluster headaches, they are probably related to your Liver.

Tension headaches, characterized by pain above the eyes, and cluster headaches, which tend to reside on the side of your head, are the most common types and should respond well to this acupressure routine. Do each point in a clockwise rotation for ten rotations and repeat three times before moving on to the next point.

Liver 2 | LV 2 is located on the foot, as described on page 179.

Liver 3 | LV 3 is located one finger-width away from LV 2, as described on page 179.

Large Intestine 4 | LI 4 is located on the hand, as described on page 179.

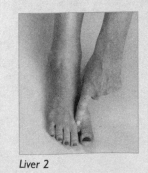

Liver 2

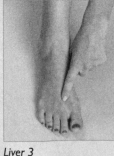

Liver 3

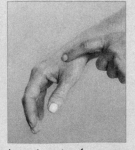

Large Intestine 4

Large Intestine 11 | Bend your elbow into your body at a 90-degree angle. LI 11 is located on the outside edge of the elbow crease.

Gallbladder 20 | GB 20 is located on the back of the neck at the base of the skull, as described on page 180.

Gallbladder 14 | GB 14 is located on the forehead, as described on page 180.

To help prevent headaches, make sure to get plenty of Liver-calming foods in your diet, especially carrots, clams, dates, oysters, plums, seaweed, spinach, and tomatoes.

In addition, drinking chrysanthemum tea is helpful because chrysanthemum sends energy to the eyes and relaxes them.

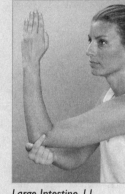
Large Intestine 11

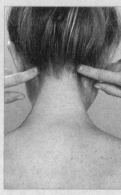
Gallbladder 20

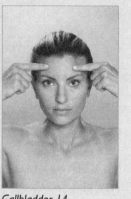
Gallbladder 14

Bladder 2 | BL 2 is located at the inside edge of your eyebrows, above the inside corner of the eyes. This point relaxes the eye area.

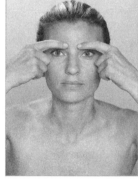
Bladder 2

The Diet Connection

When it comes to food, the Liver is finicky. Because of the Liver's influence on all of the Organs, a balanced diet is essential for the Liver type. Poor food choices will show up quickly in the way Liver types look and the way they feel. Stuart's diet was a problem because it tended to be high in fat and was too low in vegetables. He also was eating too much processed food. His drink or two after work was also a problem because the Liver and alcohol do not get along.

The Liver responds best to a clean, fresh diet. Ideally this would be an organic diet free of processed foods and preservatives. The Liver revolts against spicy-hot foods, such as curries and dishes containing chiles. Eating them in excess can harm the Liver. Fried foods also damage the Liver and should be avoided.

To keep the Liver strong and healthy, focus your diet around green vegetables, shellfish, citrus fruit, whole grains, beans, and tofu, and drink plenty of water. These foods are important in order for the Liver to properly store and circulate Qi and Blood.

Sour foods tend to calm agitated movement and are the taste associated with the fast-paced Liver. The most noteworthy in the sour category are

---

COLOR ME GREEN—WITH HEALTH

The Liver's season of strength is spring, so it is only fitting that it is partial to the color green, the color that conjures up images of foods that are fresh and healthy, such as leafy greens and other vegetables.

Nature's green foods get their coloring from chlorophyll, the substance that allows them to absorb light and convert it into energy. Chlorophyll-rich foods can improve the functions of the Liver and aid in moving Blood and Qi. The best time to eat them is when they're young plants. Lettuce and green leafy vegetables, especially spinach, are believed to be the greatest source on this chlorophyll-rich green list.

- Asparagus
- Barley grass
- Bell peppers
- Blue-green algae
- Brussels sprouts
- Celery
- Chicory
- Chives
- Collard greens
- Green beans
- Green cabbage
- Kale
- Kiwi
- Leafy greens
- Lettuce (especially romaine)
- Peas
- Seaweed
- Spinach
- Spirulina
- Swiss chard
- Turnip greens
- Wheat grass

lemons, pears, and sour plums. This is not to say that you should overdo it on these foods.

Eating a balanced diet is important for everyone, but it is crucial for Liver types because they can fall out of balance so easily. Smooth flow of Qi and Blood depends on a balanced diet! This means eating Liver-loving foods from all categories to obtain a healthy Liver, then choosing foods from all of the Organ categories.

As quickly as Liver problems tend to arise, the Liver bounces back just as quickly. Gear your diet to the Liver-friendly foods listed below and be mindful of these essential guidelines:

- Avoid alcohol in all forms.
- Avoid coffee, both regular and decaf.
- Stay away from greasy, fatty, and fried food.
- Limit your consumption of red meat to two or three times a week, and keep the serving size to four ounces or less.
- Eat spicy foods sparingly. Consider them an occasional splurge.

Foods to Balance the Liver

According to Chinese medicine, these are the foods that should be on the menus of Liver types, especially during the springtime when the Organ is most vulnerable to an imbalance.

FISH, FOWL, MEAT

These foods are important to restoring Liver Qi and Blood:

- Chicken (all parts)
- Clams
- Crab
- Cuttlefish
- Eel
- Fish (all varieties)
- Liver (organic beef and chicken liver)
- Mussels
- Oysters
- Pork (all cuts)
- Quail
- Shrimp
- Squab
- Turkey

VEGETABLES

With the Liver's affinity for the color green, vegetables are right at home. Spinach is a standout on this list.

- Alfalfa sprouts
- Asparagus
- Broccoli
- Brussels sprouts
- Cabbage
- Carrots
- Cauliflower
- Celery
- Chicory
- Cucumber
- Eggplant
- Fennel
- Leafy greens
- Leeks
- Lettuce (especially romaine)
- Mustard greens
- Onions (all varieties)
- Oyster mushrooms
- Radishes
- Scallions
- Seaweed (especially blue-green algae, kelp, and spirulina)
- Spinach
- String beans
- Tomatoes
- Watercress
- Yams

FRUIT

The Liver's affinity for the taste of sour means that the Liver diet is quite partial to fruit. In Chinese medicine, citrus is considered the most sour.

- Blackberries
- Cherries
- Citrus peel from grapefruit, lemon, lime, and orange
- Coconut
- Crabapples
- Dates
- Grapefruit
- Grapes (dark)
- Lemons
- Limes
- Loquats
- Lychees
- Kiwis
- Mangos
- Oranges
- Peaches
- Pears
- Plums (sour)
- Raspberries
- Rhubarb
- Strawberries

GRAINS

Although a number of these grains are not traditionally sour in nature, they are included to balance the Liver's influence on other Organs, particularly the Spleen and Lungs.

- Amaranth
- Barley
- Millet
- Oats
- Quinoa
- Rice (white)
- Rye
- Sprouted grains (all grains)
- Sweet rice (glutinous)
- Wheat

LEGUMES

These legumes are included to complement the Liver's influence on other Organs, particularly the Spleen and the Lungs.

- Black beans
- Black soybeans
- Mung beans
- Peas
- Tofu

NUT AND SEEDS

- Chestnuts
- Pine nuts
- Sesame seeds (especially black sesame seeds)
- Walnuts

OILS

- Black currant oil
- Coconut oil
- Flax oil
- Olive oil
- Safflower oil
- Soy oil

Tea (green, herbal, peppermint)

CONDIMENTS AND SPICES

Remember, don't overdo it when it comes to spicing your food.

- Barley malt
- Basil
- Blackstrap molasses
- Brown sugar
- Chives
- Cinnamon
- Coriander
- Cumin
- Date sugar
- Dill
- Garlic
- Ginger
- Honey
- Mint
- Mustard and mustard seeds
- Nutmeg
- Paprika
- Rosemary
- Royal jelly
- Saffron
- Stevia
- Turmeric
- Vinegar (apple cider, brown rice, and rice wine)

The Three-Day Liver Diet

This is a sample of what a typical Liver diet might look like. These menus and recipes are Liver-focused but are also designed to balance the Liver's influence on the other Organs.

DAY I

BREAKFAST

Half a grapefruit

Oatmeal with rice syrup

Chamomile tea

LUNCH

Steamed Mussels in Tomato Broth (page 188)

Salad of romaine lettuce, tomatoes, and cucumbers

Toasted whole grain bread

DINNER

Rock Cornish Game Hen Glazed with Peaches and Honey (page 190)

Sautéed string beans

Steamed brown rice

Small bowl of fresh sour cherries

DAY 2

BREAKFAST

7-grain cereal with soymilk

Whole grain rye toast with strawberry jam

Mint tea

LUNCH

Baked Ratatouille (page 190)

Steamed quinoa

Small bowl of raspberries

DINNER

Dijon White Fish Fillets (page 188)

Steamed broccoli

Baked yams

Tropical Fruit Cup (page 192)

DAY 3

BREAKFAST

Sprouted whole grain bread with sesame butter and blackberry preserves

Green tea

LUNCH

Whole wheat pasta with broccoli

Watercress and tomato salad

Baked lychees

DINNER

Sesame Baked Tofu (page 189)

Baked beets

Sautéed Spinach with Garlic and Lemon (page 191)
Plum

Rejuvenating Recipes

▩ DIJON WHITE FISH FILLETS

Fish fits the bill for the Liver type. It's nutritious and easy to digest, even oily fish such as salmon, herring, trout, and sardines. And the oils in fish are great for your skin.

4 fillets of white fish (about 6 ounces each)
2 tablespoons Dijon mustard
1 teaspoon garlic powder
½ teaspoon dried oregano
1 teaspoon sea salt
1 teaspoon freshly ground black pepper
4 sprigs parsley
1 lemon, quartered

1 Preheat the oven to 500°F and grease a 9 by 13-inch baking dish. Heat the dish in the oven for 5 minutes.

2 Rinse the fish under cold water and pat it dry with paper towels. Spread the mustard on each side of the fillets and sprinkle with the garlic powder, oregano, salt, and pepper.

3 Place the fish flat in the hot baking dish and return it to oven; bake for 10 minutes, until it turns opaque white. Garnish with the parsley and lemon quarters.

SERVES 4

▩ STEAMED MUSSELS IN TOMATO BROTH

3 pounds mussels
2 tablespoons canola oil
¼ cup minced shallots

1 8-ounce can stewed tomatoes, with their liquid
Freshly ground black pepper
½ cup chopped fresh parsley

1   Clean and debeard the mussels. Discard any that are open or broken.

2   Heat the oil in a stockpot over medium heat. Add the shallots and sauté until translucent, about 2 minutes. Stir in the stewed tomatoes with their liquid. Add the mussels. Raise heat to medium-high, cover the pot, and steam the mussels until the shells open, about 5 minutes. Pour into serving bowls, season with pepper, and garnish with the parsley.

SERVES 4

SESAME BAKED TOFU

Tofu takes on the flavor of what it is cooked with, so the ingredients give this simple-to-make entrée a distinctly Asian kick.

2 16-ounce packages firm or extra-firm tofu
⅓ cup soy sauce
¾ cup water
1 tablespoon minced fresh ginger
3 garlic cloves, minced
1½ tablespoons sesame oil
2 tablespoons sesame seeds

1   Slice each block of tofu into 4 or 5 slices and place in a shallow bowl.

2   Whisk together the soy sauce, water, ginger, garlic, and sesame oil in a medium bowl, pour the mixture over the tofu, and marinate for at least 30 minutes, up to an hour, at room temperature. Preheat the oven to 425°F. Lightly grease a baking pan.

4   Remove the tofu from the marinade, reserving the marinade, and carefully place each piece on the baking sheet. Sprinkle with the sesame seeds. Bake for 30 minutes, then rotate the sheet and drizzle with more marinade. Bake for another 15 minutes, or until the liquid has almost evaporated.

SERVES 4

◨ ROCK CORNISH GAME HEN GLAZED WITH PEACHES AND HONEY

The sweetness from the preserves and honey helps balance the Liver and the Liver's effect on the Spleen.

> 2 Cornish game hens
> ½ teaspoon sea salt
> ¼ teaspoon paprika
> 2 tablespoons unsalted butter, melted
> ¼ cup peach preserves
> 1 tablespoon honey
> 1 tablespoon grated onion
> ⅛ teaspoon ground nutmeg

1 Preheat the oven to 350°F.

2 Wash and pat dry the hens. Combine the salt and paprika and rub a third of the mixture inside the cavity of the hens. Brush 1 tablespoon of butter over the skin of the hens. Sprinkle with the remaining paprika seasoning.

3 Place the hens on a rack in a shallow baking pan and bake, uncovered, for 30 minutes.

4 While the hens are baking, combine the preserves, honey, onion, nutmeg, and the remaining 1 tablespoon butter in a small saucepan. Cook, stirring, until the preserves are melted. Brush the mixture over the hens, return them to the oven, and bake for 35 to 40 minutes longer, until golden brown and a meat thermometer reads 180°F.

5 Cover loosely and let the hens rest for 10 minutes before serving.

6 Slice the hens in half and serve.

SERVES 4

◨ BAKED RATATOUILLE

Traditionally this is a side dish, but baked in this manner it makes a nice vegetarian entrée.

2 tablespoons extra virgin olive oil

3 garlic cloves, minced

2 teaspoons dried parsley

1 eggplant, peeled and cut into ½-inch cubes

Sea salt

2 zucchini, sliced

1 large onion, sliced into rings

2 cups sliced fresh mushrooms

1 green pepper, sliced

2 large tomatoes, chopped

1   Preheat the oven to 350°F. Coat the bottom and sides of a 1½-quart casserole with 1 tablespoon of the oil.

2   Heat the remaining 1 tablespoon oil in a medium skillet over medium heat. Add the garlic and sauté about 1 minute, until lightly browned.

3   Add the parsley and eggplant and sauté until the eggplant is soft, about 10 minutes. Season with salt. Spread one layer of the eggplant evenly across the bottom of the prepared casserole dish.

4   Spread a single layer of zucchini on top of the eggplant. Season lightly with salt. Continue layering in this fashion with the onion, mushrooms, green pepper, and tomatoes until all the vegetables are added, ending with a layer of eggplant. Bake for 45 minutes, until tender to the touch with a fork.

SERVES 4

SAUTÉED SPINACH WITH GARLIC AND LEMON

Spinach is one of the best foods you can eat for the Liver. This easy preparation takes advantage of other Liver-friendly ingredients.

3 pounds fresh baby spinach

3 tablespoons canola oil

3 garlic cloves, peeled

Juice of 1 large lemon

Sea salt and freshly ground black pepper

1 Wash and dry the spinach leaves. Heat the oil in a large skillet over medium heat. Add the whole garlic and sauté until it starts to soften and become translucent, about 5 minutes.

2 Add the spinach to the pan a handful at a time. As it starts to wilt, add another handful until it all fits in the pan, stirring frequently. Add the lemon juice and season with salt and pepper and continue to cook for 2 minutes. Serve hot.

SERVES 4

▨ TROPICAL FRUIT CUP

1 cup halved seedless dark grapes
2 kiwis, peeled and cut into cubes
1 large mango, peeled, seeded, and cut into cubes
1 lemon
2 tablespoons brown sugar
4 fresh cherries
4 fresh mint leaves

1 Combine the grapes, kiwis, and mango in a large bowl. Cut the lemon in half and squeeze the juice over the fruit. Add the brown sugar and stir. Refrigerate for 30 minutes.

2 Divide the fruit into 4 parfait glasses and top each with a cherry and a mint leaf.

SERVES 4

Self-Care for Livery Skin

Western and Chinese medicine agree that a balanced diet, a good night's sleep, relaxation, exercise, and avoiding sun damage are key for staying healthy and combating wrinkles. Eastern medicine also touts the benefits of the goji berry, a fruit particularly high in vitamin E that is found in China and the Himalayas. You can eat dried goji berries or drink the berries as a juice.

The primary skin care ingredients for combating wrinkles are vitamins A, C, E, and D. Vitamin A (retinol) is said to stimulate the production

9-1-1 RESCUE THERAPY: SUNSPOTS

Whether you call them liver spots, sunspots, or age spots, they're all the same thing: unsightly but benign brown patches that form as extra pigment in the skin and can show up on the face, hands, shoulders, arms, forehead, and bald scalp.

Western medicine claims they are all but impossible to get rid of without going to extremes, such as laser treatment, cryotherapy (cold therapy), or chemical peels. Chinese medicine says the way to get rid of them is by getting Liver Blood moving properly. This is an acupressure routine that can make it happen. It can also be used after pregnancy by women who develop melasma, discolored patches that can appear on the face during pregnancy and are commonly called "the mask of pregnancy."

Do the entire routine three times.

Liver 3 | LV 3 is located on the top of your foot, between the web of the first and second toe.

Spleen 6 | SP 6 is located on the inside of the leg, roughly four finger-widths above the top of the ankle bone.

Spleen 10 | Place the palm of your hand on the bottom of your opposite knee with the thumb extended upward. Your thumb should fall on SP 10, located about three finger-widths above the inside of the knee.

Large Intestine 11 | Bend your elbow into your body at a 90-degree angle. LI 11 is located at the elbow on the outside edge of the crease.

Then massage the spots with the following pearl powder formula.

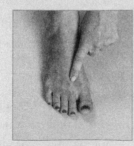

Liver 3

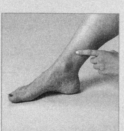

Spleen 6

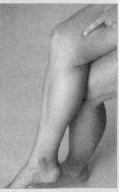

Spleen 10

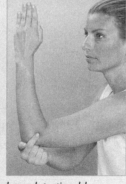

Large Intestine 11

OUT, OUT, LIVER SPOT

Pearl powder, which is ground mother-of-pearl, is commonly used in Chinese medicine as a natural anti-inflammatory and detoxifier. It was the ancient secret used among the Chinese empresses for wrinkle-free skin. Today it is commonly found in Asian skin-care formulas to combat the signs of wrinkles. When combined with safflower oil, it evens skin coloring and lightens sunspots.

I dime-size pinch pearl powder
½ teaspoon safflower oil

Mix the pearl powder with the safflower oil to form a paste. Massage the paste into the sunspots for 15 seconds and rinse off with tepid water. Do this twice a day for 30 days.

In addition, you can add these Liver-friendly foods to your diet:

- Cucumbers
- Fish of all kinds
- Green leafy vegetables
- Pine nuts
- Sesame seeds (especially black)
- Tomatoes
- Walnuts

of collagen. Vitamin C (ascorbic acid) is a powerful antioxidant and anti-inflammatory, and vitamin E (tocopherol) is also used to reduce inflammation and smooth skin texture. Studies have shown that vitamin D supplements help skin to maintain moisture.

To combat fine lines, reverse the impact of environmental damage, and prevent further skin wrinkling, look for all-natural, organic skin creams that utilize vitamins A, C, and E. Most oils, particularly jojoba and avocado, are high in vitamins A and E. Grapefruit, orange, lemon, and other natural fruits and fruit acids are rich in vitamin C. Anti-wrinkle and complexion-evening products can be applied all over your face at night and as a spot treatment underneath your day cream.

Remember, the Liver is more affected by stress than any other Organ, so taking the time to relax is one of the most effective cures for Livery skin. Increase or decrease the ingredient proportions to suit your desired consistency or result. Before using any product, whether homemade or purchased, I recommend performing a skin allergy patch test (page 219).

TIME-OUT CURE

You can use this in combination with any of the treatments in this chapter or apply it to your skin whenever you feel stressed or worn. It relaxes not just your skin but your whole body as well. It is perfect as a night oil or as a spot treatment during the day.

> **2 ounces almond oil**
> **2 drops jasmine essential oil**
> **2 drops rose essential oil**

1 Combine the almond oil and essential oils in a small, clean dark or amber glass jar with a tight-fitting lid.

2 Put a few drops of the blended oil on your hand and rub your hands together gently to warm the oil. Cup your hands over your nose and take 3 deep breaths.

3 Put your hands on your cheeks and sweep downward from your face to the top of your neck outward across your décolleté to your shoulder.

4 Take another deep breath and relax.

AVOCADO DELIGHT TREATMENT MASK

Avocado is an excellent ingredient for reducing wrinkles and moisturizing dry skin. In this formula, the honey tightens the pores, while safflower oil and spearmint even skin coloring. This mask is intended to be applied to the wrinkles but can be applied as a mask to the full face.

> **Flesh of ¼ very ripe avocado**
> **1 teaspoon safflower oil**

2 tablespoons crushed spearmint leaves

I teaspoon honey

1 Combine the ingredients in a blender and blend until creamy, about 30 seconds.

2 Apply to affected areas and leave overnight. In the morning, remove with warm water and continue with your skin care regime.

3 If using as a full face mask, remove after 20 minutes, rinse with warm water, and apply your favorite face cream.

▦ SWEET ORANGE WRINKLE MINIMIZER

Sweet orange and rose essential oils are known for their effectiveness at reducing the appearance of wrinkles. Almond oil is a light oil that helps essential oils get quickly absorbed into your skin. Coconut oil rehydrates your skin and seals in skin moisture. White flower oil soothes your muscles and relaxes your mind. Use it alone at night. During the day, apply to affected areas and wait until it is absorbed into your skin (about 10 minutes) before applying day cream.

2 tablespoons almond oil

2 tablespoons coconut oil (cooking oil)

½ teaspoon white flower oil

8 drops sweet orange essential oil

8 drops rose essential oil

1 Place the almond and coconut oils in a small, clean dark or amber-colored glass bottle. Add the white flower oil and the orange and rose essential oils.

2 Morning and night, massage a few drops into your face after washing it.

IF YOU DON'T WANT TO MAKE IT, THEN BUY IT . . .

Treatment products, whether serums or creams, can be expensive but are well worth the price. They generally target a specific issue, such as wrinkles or sunspots. I've found these natural products to be very effective.

Yon-Ka Paris Mesonium

Cost: About $76

Size: 1 oz.

This product consists of two synergetic concentrates. Its exceptional concentration of essential all-plant amino acids produces rejuvenating activity deep in the skin. It combats free radicals and reduces the appearance of fine lines and wrinkles.

Dr. Hauschka Regenerating Serum

Cost: About $85

Size: 1 oz.

This activating serum firms skin and minimizes the appearance of fine lines and wrinkles. Antioxidant-rich red clover helps stimulate the production of healthy skin cells, while hydrating quince seed extract, revitalizing kalanchoe extract, and organic clover blossom honey help support the skin's natural health and renewal.

Naturopathica Primrose Eye and Upper Lip Treatment Cream

Cost: Around $48

Size: .5 oz.

This cream is designed to soothe and smooth dry and wrinkled skin around eyes and lips. It is a nourishing blend of rich evening primrose oil, which is high in skin-softening gamma linolenic acid, and açaí fruit oil, a moisturizer.

Naturopathica Botanical Skin Brightener

Cost: Around $68

Size: 2.5 oz.

This brightening cream contains skin-lightening licorice extract to reduce the appearance of sunspots; kojic acid, a mushroom-derived ingredient, to inhibit further production of sunspot development; and lactic acid derived from yogurt to smooth the skin's surface.

10

Feeding Your Face the *Right* Way

the desert of Morocco, I frequently would be served warm peppermint tea with a lot of sugar. I could not understand why people drank hot beverages in blistering weather. Had I focused less on what I thought and more on how I felt, I would have noticed that although the temperature of my tea was warm, it actually made me feel cool.

According to Chinese medicine, peppermint has a Yin property. This means that when consumed, it produces a Yin-like effect in your body. It reduces heat, hydrates you, and cools you down. Sugar also is Yin, and when it is taken with peppermint, the Yin characteristics of both are enhanced. So next time you are running around in the heat of the summer without water, a cup of hot peppermint tea (you don't need the sugar) instead of a cold soda not only will relieve your thirst, but will make you feel cooler. And it is healthier for you. It is one of the many lessons from the vast sea of knowledge that is Chinese medicine.

As you now know from reading this book, how you feed your body plays a central role in the quality of your appearance, as well as your overall health. Chinese medicine does not recognize a difference between internal health and external beauty. They exist as one. The quality of this existence—your Qi, Blood, Essence, and Organs—is dependent on the nourishment it receives. Nourishment comes from varied sources, including the air you breathe and the lifestyle you lead, but it comes foremost from the quality of the food and beverages you consume. As far as Chinese medicine is concerned, you truly are what you eat.

The key to eating right for your appearance and your overall health is *balance*. The idea of a balanced diet differs between Eastern and Western philosophies. In chapters 5 through 9 you learned about the foods that complement your Organ type. These are your foods of focus. You should concentrate on eating more of them when your Organ is out of harmony and during the season in which you are most vulnerable to an Organ imbalance. You should turn to them when you're emotionally edgy or have digestion problems. By the same token, if you are feeling an imbalance in another Organ, you should be turning to the foods that complement that Organ type, in addition to eating your own Organ foods.

When you are in a state of balance, you maintain balance by eating from the variety of foods that complement all the Organs and by concentrating on getting both Yin and Yang foods in your meals. When you dine at a traditional Chinese restaurant, notice the variety of foods on your plate. They are selected for taste, texture, temperature, and color—balance. You'll also be served, or at least offered, hot tea. The Chinese have almost a sixth sense for balancing food.

I admit, it isn't easy. Mastering food selection in today's fast-paced world, where so much of our food contains artificial ingredients, is nearly impossible. All we can try to do is strive for balance. To this end, on page 204 you will find a master chart that includes foods common to an American diet. It tells you whether a food is Yin or Yang (or both), the Organ or Organs it nourishes and the Meridian entered, its taste, and its temperature. You can also use this chart to select foods that address a specific cosmetic concern or health problem. There may be minor discrepancies between this chart and others, as even practitioners of Chinese medicine often find it difficult to distinguish the subtle medicinal effects of certain foods.

If it helps, think of achieving a perfect day of weather inside your body.

Mild temperature, sunny skies, and clean air should always be your goal! The food you consume will affect the balance of your body's weather system. If it's hot, humid, and muggy, you certainly will feel soggy, limp, and tired. You should be eating foods that are cooling and flow out of the body. When it is cold outside, your internal temperature is going to feel the discomfort, so you want to eat warming foods that move inward to the body.

These are guidelines to help you use the chart:

Yin and Yang. A balanced diet is one that is not too Yin and not too Yang. Unfortunately, it is not that black and white. In winter, the most Yin season, you want to eat more Yang foods, and in summer, the most Yang season, you'll want to eat more Yin foods. When you have a Yang deficiency, you need more Yang foods, and when you have a Yin deficiency, you need more Yin foods. Your state of health and the season play strongly into the balance of Yin and Yang.

Categories. This chart divides foods in categories for a reason. Meats, though not all, tend to be mostly Yang, and fruits, though not all, tend to be mostly Yin. Legumes tend to be more Yin. Grains are Yin and Yang. This is why eating a variety of foods from all food groups is important.

Deciding which category to eat from when you have an Organ imbalance can be a little tricky, however. For example, if you have a Spleen imbalance, simply supplementing your diet with Spleen-strengthening foods will help. But if the reason the Spleen is weak is that the Liver is too strong, then eating Spleen-strengthening foods is like bailing water from a leaky boat with a bucket instead of trying to stop the leak. Eventually you're going to sink. The "leak" is the Liver. When the Liver is too strong, it hinders the Spleen and prevents it from performing optimally. So you need to fortify the Spleen by sedating the Liver, meaning you should eat both Liver-calming and Spleen-strengthening foods.

Temperature. Balancing your diet relates not only to your Organ type but also to your physical constitution. In the Chinese diet, there are six types of physical constitutions. As with everything else, most people lean toward one, even though they can be a combination of two or more. For example, you can have the emotional attributes and physique of a Heart type but be cold instead of hot, which is typical of the Heart. Then there are times when your dietary needs run counter to your physical constitution. If you have a

9-1-1 RESCUE THERAPY: INDIGESTION

If you are under a lot of stress and have indigestion or a stomachache, your Liver could be invading your Spleen. If this is the case, cook foods from the Spleen and Liver category. These are ideal choices:

- Basil
- Beans (red and black)
- Caraway seeds
- Chicken
- Coconut meat
- Dates
- Dill seeds
- Eggplant
- Garlic
- Mustard seeds
- Oregano
- Saffron
- Spearmint tea
- Sweet potatoes
- Sweet rice
- Tofu
- White rice

cold constitution, when you're sick with the flu or you have a fever, then you may temporarily need to eat cold foods, no matter what your Organ type. Figuring out your internal temperature isn't as difficult as it may seem if you follow these basic guidelines.

Hot. Your internal temperature runs hot if you have a reddish complexion, get frequent skin eruptions, and frequently feel hot and/or thirsty. If this sounds like you, eat cooling foods.

Cold. Your internal temperature is cold if you have a whitish, pale complexion and frequently feel cold when others are warm, especially when it's hot outside. If this sounds like you, eat warming foods.

Dry. People prone to internal dryness have dry skin, lips, and mucous membranes in the nose. They also are often thirsty. They tend to be thin and have difficulty gaining weight. If this sounds like you, eat moistening foods.

Damp. People prone to dampness look puffy in the face and middle and feel heavy, sluggish, and tired. They can have difficulty losing weight. If this sounds like you, eat drying foods.

Deficiency. This is characterized by a pale complexion, fatigue, shortness of breath, and underweight. If this sounds like you, you should eat Yang foods.

Excess in any Organ. This is characterized by a reddish complexion, lots of energy or hyperactivity, and possibly greater than average physical strength. If this sounds like you, you should eat Yin foods.

Organ/Meridian. Certain foods have a natural affinity for specific Organs. As you've learned, when a certain food is eaten, the Spleen sorts the good nourishment from the bad and sends it out through the body in the form of Qi. The nourishment, depending on what it is, travels to a specific Organ or Organs. Most foods have a kinship with more than one Organ. When you have a deficiency related to a specific Organ, you want to eat more of these Organ foods.

Taste/flavor. Balance comes from eating a meal composed of all five tastes: bitter, salty, sour, spicy, and sweet. The ratio in which you combine these tastes can change according to the season of the year and your individual needs.

As you learned in Chapter 2, a food's flavor also influences certain Organs. Sweet-tasting foods complement the Spleen, sour foods complement the Liver, bitter foods complement the Heart, salty foods affect the Kidneys, and spicy, or pungent, foods affect the Lungs.

Temperature/movement. As I illustrated at the beginning of this chapter, food has an effect on your internal temperature. Under normal circumstances, you should eat warming foods in the winter and cooling foods in the summer. The taste of a food warms or cools by sending its energy to an area of your body. Warm and hot foods have a spicy taste and move upward or outward. Cool or cold foods have a sour, salty, or bitter taste and move downward or inward. Sweet foods can be cool or warm.

Here are other guidelines, based on principles of Chinese medicine, to help you in food selection and preparation:

Tip the balance with cooking methods. You can make foods more Yang (warming) with these methods:

- Baking
- Deep-frying (though this is not generally recommended)
- Roasting
- Stir-frying

You can make your food more Yin (cooling) by:

- Boiling
- Poaching
- Steaming

Moderation is balance. Think of that plate in an upscale traditional Chinese restaurant. There is a nice balance in the variety of protein, vegetables, and grains. Not too heavy in anything. Moderation also applies to the amount of food you eat. Eat only until you are satisfied, not until you are full.

Be aware of what you're eating. This means paying attention to your food and eating it slowly. Pay attention to the texture, appreciate the tastes. Feel the temperature, which is so important to maintaining balance. Notice the subtlety of sweet, sour, bitter, spicy, salty. Taste is important because the primary taste sends nutrition to the corresponding organ. Eating with intent also aids digestion. The more you learn about Chinese diet, the easier it will be to apply it.

THE NOURISHING QUALITIES OF FOOD

FOOD	YIN	YANG	ORGANS/MERIDIANS	TEMPERATURE	FLAVOR	EFFECTS
Fish						
Anchovy		x	SP, ST	neutral	sweet	lifts and tones sagging muscles, decreases facial swelling
Catfish	x	x	SP, ST	neutral	sweet	nourishes muscles, regulates digestion
Clam	x		LV, K	cold	sweet, salty	softens wrinkles, improves vision and hearing
Crab	x		LV	cold	salty	softens wrinkles, lightens sunspots
Herring		x	SP, L	neutral	sweet	regulates pores, drains facial puffiness
Mussel	x	x	LV, K	warm	salty	sharpens memory hearing and vision
Oyster	x		LV	neutral	sweet, salty	moistens skin and nails
Shrimp	x	x	LV, K	slightly warm	sweet	thickens hair, moistens tendons and ligaments
Tuna	x	x	K, ST	neutral	sweet, salty	drains undereye and facial puffiness, lifts jowls
White fish		x	SP, L, LV, ST	neutral	sweet	tones facial muscles, regulates pores, softens wrinkles
Fowl						
Chicken		x	SP, ST	warm	sweet	nourishes and tones facial muscles
Chicken (egg)	x	x	SP, K	neutral	sweet	decreases undereye and facial puffiness, thickens hair
Duck	x	x	SP, L, K	neutral	sweet, salty	lifts jowls, lifts sagging muscles, strengthens bones
Goose	x		SP, L	neutral	sweet	heals bruises, regulates hair moisture
Turkey	x		SP, ST	warm	sweet	tones muscles, regulates digestion
Meat						
Beef	x		SP, ST, LI	warm	sweet	tones muscles, regulates digestion
Lamb		x	SP, K	warm	sweet	tones facial muscles, drains facial puffiness
Pork	x		SP, K, ST	neutral	sweet, salty	builds muscles, moistens lips
Rabbit	x	x	SP, ST, LI	cool	sweet	nourishes muscles, clears sinus congestion
Vegetables						
Asparagus	x		L, K	cold	sweet	thickens hair, strengthens teeth and bones
Cabbage		x	SP, ST	neutral	sweet	heals bruises, decreases swelling
Carrot	x	x	SP, LV, L	neutral	sweet	lifts jowls, improves vision, lubricates intestines
Celery	x		LV, ST, BL	cool	sweet	softens wrinkles, clears hot skin eruptions
Corn		x	ST, LI	neutral	sweet	tones muscles, regulates pores
Cucumber	x		ST, BL	cool	sweet	reduces breakouts, clears and evens complexion
Eggplant	x		ST, LI	slightly cold	sweet	lifts jowls, heals bruises
Fennel		x	SP, LV, ST	neutral/raw, warm/cooked	sweet	lifts sagging muscles, moistens tendons and ligaments

Vegetable			Organs	Flavor	Temperature	Effects
Lettuce	×		ST, LI	sweet, bitter	cool	strengthens muscle tone, balances combination skin
Mushroom	×		SP, L, ST, LI	sweet	slightly cold	relieves sinus congestion, decreases swelling, drains hot skin eruptions
Onion	×	×	SP, L, ST, LI	spicy, bitter	warm	strengthens muscle tone, balances combination skin, clears sinus congestion
Pea	×	×	SP, ST	sweet	neutral	decreases facial swelling, dries pimples
Potato (sweet)	×		SP, K, ST,	sweet	neutral	moistens lips and dry skin
Potato (white)		×	SP, ST	sweet	neutral	decreases swelling, regulates digestion
Radish	×	×	L, ST	sweet, spicy	cool	regulates pores, clears outbreaks
Seaweed (kelp)	×		LV, L, K, ST	salty	cold	softens wrinkles, strengthens hair, decreases undereye puffiness and redness
Spinach	×		LV, ST, LI	sweet	cool	prevents wrinkles, strengthens muscle tone, moistens skin and nails
String bean		×	SP, K	sweet	neutral	regulates facial fluid metabolism
Turnip	×		L, ST	sweet, spicy	cool	relieves facial congestion, lubricates intestines
Watercress	×	×	L, ST	sweet, spicy	cool	moistens dry skin, regulates pores
Yam		×	SP, L, K	sweet	neutral	regulates facial fluid metabolism, reduces jowls, evens complexion

Fruit

Fruit			Organs	Flavor	Temperature	Effects
Apple	×	×	SP, ST	sweet, sour	cool	clears breakouts around mouth, tones muscles
Apricot	×		L, ST	sweet, sour	cool	balances complexion, heals bruises
Banana	×		ST, LI	sweet	cool	clears hot skin eruptions, tones muscles
Cherry		×	SP, LV, K	sweet, sour	warm	strengthens muscles, softens wrinkles, lifts jowls
Grape	×	×	ST, LV, K	sweet, sour	neutral	improves vision and hearing, drains puffiness
Grapefruit	×		L, ST	sour	cold	regulates pores, drains facial toxins
Lemon	×		ST, LV, L	sour	cold	regulates skin moisture, softens wrinkles
Mango	×	×	SP, LV	sweet, sour	cold	lifts sagging muscles, decreases muscle tension
Mulberry	×	×	LV, K	sweet	cool	lightens sunspots, sharpens memory
Olive	×	×	L, ST	sweet, sour	neutral	evens skin moisture and coloring
Orange	×		ST, BL	sweet, sour	cool	minimizes bruises, reduces undereye darkness
Papaya	×	×	SP, HT	sweet, bitter	neutral	minimizes broken capillaries and bruises
Peach	×	×	ST, LI	sweet, sour	neutral	moistens hair, improves muscle tone
Pear	×		L, ST	sweet, sour	cool	regulates pores, tones muscles
Persimmon	×		L, HT, LI	sweet	cold	regulates pores, evens blotchy skin
Pineapple	×		ST, BL	sweet, sour	slightly cold	reduces hot skin eruptions, drains puffiness
Plum	×		LV, ST	sweet, sour	cold	softens wrinkles, lifts jowls
Raspberry	×	×	SP, LV	sweet	neutral	nourishes facial muscles, improves vision
Strawberry	×	×	LV, K	sweet, sour	warm	moistens tendons and ligaments, strengthens bones

FOOD	YIN	YANG	ORGANS/MERIDIANS	TEMPERATURE	FLAVOR	EFFECTS
Fruit						
Tangerine	x		L, ST	slightly cool	sweet, sour	relieves sinus congestion, lubricates intestines
Tomato	x		LV, ST	cool	sweet, sour	minimizes sunspots, evens facial coloring
Watermelon	x		HT, ST, BL	cold	sweet	evens blotchy skin, decreases swelling
Grains						
Barley	x		SP, ST, BL	slightly cold	sweet, salty	tones muscles, decreases swelling
Buckwheat (kasha)	x	x	SP, ST, LI	cool	sweet	improves muscle tone, drains puffiness
Corn		x	ST, BL	neutral	sweet	regulates digestion, moistens dry skin
Millet	x		SP, K, ST	slightly cold	sweet, slightly salty	evens skin coloring, sharpens memory
Rice (brown)		x	SP, ST, LI	neutral	sweet	tones muscles, lifts jowls
Rice (glutinous, sweet)		x	SP, L, ST	warm	sweet	regulates body temperature, evens skin coloring
Rice (white)		x	SP, ST	neutral	sweet	sculpts jawline, cheeks, and neck
Rye	x		LI, SI	slightly cold	sweet	minimizes broken capillaries, regulates fluid metabolism
Wheat (whole wheat flour)	x	x	SP, HT, K	cool	sweet	reduces spider veins, decreases undereye and facial puffiness
Wheat (white flour)	x		SP, HT, K	cool	sweet	moistens lips, clears redness, moistens withered skin
Legumes						
Adzuki bean	x		HT, SI	neutral	sweet, sour	clears redness, reduces anxiety
Kidney bean	x		SP, LI, SI	neutral	sweet	reduces facial puffiness and clears sinus congestion
Mung bean	x		HT, ST	cool	sweet	decreases swelling and bloating
Soybean	x	x	SP, LI	cool	sweet	lifts jowls, clears hot skin eruptions
Soybean (tofu)	x	x	L, ST, LI	cool	sweet	regulates hair moisture, reduces eye redness
Nuts, Seeds						
Almond		x	L	neutral	sweet	evens and balances complexion
Chestnut		x	SP, K	warm	sweet	drains facial puffiness
Pine nut	x	x	L, LV, LI	slightly warm	sweet	moistens dry skin and nails, relieves constipation
Peanut		x	SP, L	neutral	sweet	clears facial and sinus congestion
Sesame seed (black)		x	LV, K	neutral	sweet	thickens and nourishes hair
Sunflower seed		x	L, LI	warm	sweet	regulates pores, relieves constipation
Walnut	x	x	L, K	warm	sweet	strengthens and thickens hair
Oils						
Peanut	x	x	L, ST	cool	sweet	evens combination skin
Safflower		x	HT, LV	warm	spicy	minimizes spider veins, relieves headaches

	x1	x2	x3	Meridian	Temp	Flavor	Benefits
Sesame	x	x		ST	cool	sweet	moistens dry skin and lips
Soy	x	x		ST, LI	hot	sweet, spicy	regulates skin moisture, clears redness

Dairy and Soy

	x1	x2	x3	Meridian	Temp	Flavor	Benefits
Butter		x		SP, ST, LI	warm	sweet	nourishes and tones facial muscles, lifts sagging muscles
Cheese (cow's milk)	x			L, HT, ST	neutral	sweet	brightens complexion, regulates pores
Cheese (sheep milk)	x	x		SP, K	warm	sweet	decreases undereye and facial puffiness
Milk/Yogurt (cow's milk)	x			SP, L, HT	neutral	sweet	moistens lips, regulates pores, evens complexion
Milk/Yogurt (soy)	x			SP, L, ST	cool	sweet	tones facial muscles, reduces sinus congestion

Beverages

	x1	x2	x3	Meridian	Temp	Flavor	Benefits
Alcohol	x			LV, L, HT, ST	warm	sweet, bitter	increases circulation
Beer	x			K, HT	warm	sweet, bitter	increases circulation
Coffee	x			HT	warm	sweet, bitter	in moderation, improves mental clarity, increases circulation
Tea	x			LV, HT, ST, LI, BL	cool	sweet, slightly bitter	in moderation, improves mental clarity
Wine	x			LV, HT, L, ST	warm	sweet, bitter	increases circulation

Condiments/Spices

	x1	x2	x3	Meridian	Temp	Flavor	Benefits
Basil	x			SP, ST	warm	spicy	tones muscles, heals bruises
Bay leaf	x			L	warm	spicy	regulates hair moisture
Cinnamon	x			SP, K, BL	hot	spicy	moistens lips, brightens under eyes
Dill	x			SP, K	warm	spicy	decreases facial and undereye puffiness, lifts jowls
Garlic	x			SP, L, ST	warm	sweet, spicy	regulates pores and clears congestion
Ginger	x			SP, L, ST	hot	spicy	moistens dry skin and lips, lifts jowls
Honey	x	x		SP, L, LI	neutral	sweet	brightens complexion, regulates pores
Maltose	x	x		SP, L, ST	warm	sweet	in moderation, strengthens muscle tore
Mustard		x		SP, L, ST	warm	spicy	nourishes facial muscles, moistens dry skin, lubricates intestines
Nutmeg		x		SP, LI	warm	spicy	lifts sagging muscles, lifts jowls
Pepper (black)	x			SP, ST, LI	hot	spicy	strengthens muscles, dries oily skin
Pepper (cayenne)	x			HT, SP, ST	hot	spicy	clears redness, minimizes spider veins
Peppermint	x	x		L, HT, LI	cold	sweet	balances combination skin, minimizes broken capillaries
Rosemary		x		L	warm	spicy	reduces headache, reverses premature balding
Salt	x			K, ST, LI, SI	cold	salty	improves hearing, soothes sore throat
Spearmint		x		SP, L	warm	sweet, spicy	balances combination skin, lifts jowls
Sugar (brown)	x			SP, LV, ST	warm	sweet	in moderation, tightens muscles, relieves stomach pain
Sugar (white)	x			SP, L, ST	neutral	sweet	in moderation, moisturizes skin
Vinegar	x			LV, ST	neutral	sweet, sour	minimizes sunspots, evens skin coloring

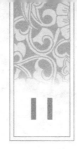

Skin Care Rituals for a Fit Face

IN A PERFECT WORLD, WE'D ALL HAVE PERFECT skin—a soft rosy complexion, fine pores, even skin tone, and a radiant silky appearance. Perfect skin is normal skin. Our Western culture believes that we are all born with a skin *type,* which may or may not be normal. Life's circumstances, such as your health, age, diet, hormones, lifestyle, and too much sun exposure can affect your skin type, causing a less-than-perfect skin *condition*. Chinese medicine says we are all born with normal skin, and changes occur when we are not in balance. Earlier in this book you learned how that happens. Nevertheless, normal skin is not normal for most of us.

Western and Eastern medicine agree that your face consists of three layers of skin cells:

- The **epidermis** is the outer coating of the skin and what's visible to the eye. It is covered by a protective coating known as the acid mantle, a thin, oily film with an ideal pH level of 4.5 to 5.5.

- The middle layer, or stratum, is the **dermis**. It contains collagen, the substance that gives skin its volume, and elastin, which gives skin its elasticity. The quality of the living cells in this layer determines the skin's health. Blood vessels, oil glands, nerve fibers, hair follicles, and sweat glands are located in the dermis.
- The bottom layer is called the **subcutaneous** layer. It is primarily made up of fat and determines the plumpness of your face. In Chinese medicine, this layer also houses your muscles.

Cell growth starts at the bottom of the dermal layer and travels upward to the epidermis. As cells migrate to the top, they use up their nutrients, lose their vitality, their water content diminishes, and they die. It is why the texture and suppleness of your skin change as you get older.

Western philosophy leads us to believe that as you age, your skin thins and becomes more fragile, pore size shrinks, and your skin naturally starts to dry. As it loses its plumpness and elasticity, muscle tone weakens and the skin starts to sag. You also develop wrinkles. Before reading this book you may have thought that unless drastic measures were taken, your beauty days were over. Now you know this is not true.

PH AND WHAT IT MEANS

The term pH stands for the "potential of hydrogen," or what is commonly referred to as an acid or alkaline level. Numbers lower than 7 measure the degree of acidity, while numbers higher than 7 rank the level of alkalinity. The lower the number, the greater the acidity. The higher the number, the greater the alkalinity. A value of 7 is neutral—equal parts of both.

Optimum pH values in the body depend upon the function being performed. For example, the pH of the stomach is very acidic, around 1, because stomach acids are necessary to break down the foods we eat. The acid mantle of your skin is slightly acidic (4.5 to 5.5) in order to fight off harmful bacteria. Foaming face wash, particularly soap, can be highly alkaline, up to pH 12. Although washing your face with foamy soap leaves your skin feeling squeaky clean, what you experience when your skin squeaks is the absence of your protective acid mantle.

What's Your Skin Type?

How your skin ages depends on the way you treat it—its exposure to the elements, especially the sun, and how you cleanse and pamper it. No one can dispute this. But as you have learned, the quality of your skin depends a great deal on the quality of your health. Both Western and Eastern skin experts recognize five skin types:

Normal—Normal skin looks dewy and is as soft as a baby's behind. It is rosy, blemish-free, even textured, and feels smooth to the touch. The acid mantle is at the ideal pH range of 4.5 to 5.5.

Oily—Oily skin looks shiny, greasy, and wet. It is characterized by large pores, which means a greater-than-average production of oil. Due to its higher oil content, this type of skin, although less prone to wrinkles, is more prone to blemishes and acne. People with oily skin tend to wash their face frequently to "get rid" of the oil. However, frequent washing can irritate skin, strip the acid mantle, and trick your oil glands into secreting more oil. All of which increases your chance of attracting bacteria and getting pimples.

Dry—Dry skin looks dry, dull, and lifeless. There are two types of dry skin—oil-dry and water-dry. When you have oil-dry skin, you have small pores that produce a limited amount of oil. Water-dry skin has less to do with pore size and more to do with drinking enough water, avoiding nicotine, not eating too much spicy or salty food, minimizing your caffeine and alcohol intake, and increasing your water consumption if you take diuretics or after a sweaty workout. When your skin is water-dry, your body needs more water, no matter what your pore size. Although less prone to breakouts, both types of dry skin are prone to premature aging, fine lines, and wrinkles.

Combination—Combination skin is characterized by having two or more types of skin. It is commonly seen as an oily T-zone, with a shiny nose, forehead, and chin, and dryness (oil or water) on the cheeks and sides of the forehead. With combination skin, breakouts occur in the oily areas and fine lines and wrinkles develop in the dry areas.

Sensitive—Sensitive skin tends to be highly reactive. It is easily irritated, turns red for no apparent reason, and can break out, itch, or flake. This type of skin is prone to redness, blemishes, sudden outbreaks, irritation, some forms of rosacea, and patches of dryness. In Western medicine, it is considered a skin type and a skin condition. In Chinese medicine, it is considered a skin condition.

"Conditions" Change

A skin *condition* is different from skin *type*. Both Western and Chinese medicines agree that a skin condition is something we acquire. Blemishes, acne, redness, rashes, rosacea, dryness, and pallor are just the short list of skin conditions that you can acquire. Although skin problems manifest externally, in Chinese medicine their root causes involve internal imbalances between Yin, Yang, Qi, Blood, and Organs. The six external environmental evils can also instigate a skin problem.

A skin care regime that nourishes your skin will accentuate what you set out to achieve with the AcuFacial® Acupressure Facelift and other acupressure massages you choose.

How to Care for Your Skin

Rituals provide meaning and structure to our lives. Often life becomes so harried and overwhelming that we let go of the daily rituals that make us feel and look better. Though exercise is commonly noted as "the first thing to

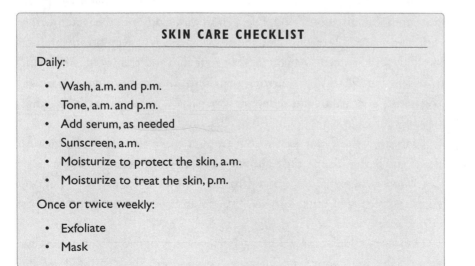

SKIN CARE CHECKLIST

Daily:

- Wash, a.m. and p.m.
- Tone, a.m. and p.m.
- Add serum, as needed
- Sunscreen, a.m.
- Moisturize to protect the skin, a.m.
- Moisturize to treat the skin, p.m.

Once or twice weekly:

- Exfoliate
- Mask

go" when life overwhelms, this is usually not the case. It's skin care, especially among women.

Women are often conditioned to take care of others first—it's a common trait that is often taken to the extreme among Spleen types. We feel "vanity" cannot supersede getting the kids out of bed and off to school or fixing lunches the night before. In the morning there isn't enough time, and at night we're too tired. But is this *balance*? Of course not!

As you've learned from this book, balance is the secret to perpetual youth—in the way you look, the way you feel, and the way you act. Chinese medicine is based on the concept of balance. When you take the time to attend to your skin care needs, it is not vanity. It is value. You are valuing yourself and your health. It takes no more than a few minutes in the morning and a few minutes before you go to bed to calm, cleanse, tone, and moisturize your face. It's the finishing touch that will help give you your best face now, no matter what your age. So indulge and enjoy.

Daily Rituals

You *can* and should begin and end each day with a pause—just a moment to stop and breathe. That's all you need to take in and let go of the things that stop you from being your beautiful, balanced you.

Wake up and relax. Begin and end each day by placing three drops of your favorite essential oil in a bowl or sink filled with warm water. Swirl the water around to disperse the oil. Dip a clean washcloth into the water, wring it out, and place it over your face and neck. Take a few deep breaths, filling your body with its scent. As you awaken your skin and relax your mind, you are also hydrating and moisturizing your skin. In the morning, choose an invigorating essential oil like lemon or rosemary. Wind down in the evening by using calming essential oils such as chamomile or lavender.

Cleanse. Wash your face with a cleanser that's right for your type of skin. If you haven't found the right one yet, here are your options:

Creamy cleansers are liquid and have a milky color and feel. They are designed to gently clean and hydrate your skin. They are good for normal, dry, and sensitive skin.

Gel cleansers look and feel like gel. They are designed to remove excess oil and debris from your skin. They are translucent or slightly tinted. When

you wash your face with them, they foam. Gel cleansers are good for oily or acne skin. Don't overdo it, though, or you will strip your valuable acid mantle.

Soaps come in liquid or bar form. Super-fatted soaps contain fatty substances, such as cocoa butter, lanolin, or cold cream to oil and hydrate dry skin. Acne soaps often contain salicylic acid, tea tree oil, or some form of antibacterial ingredient. Beauty bars and transparent soaps come in many varieties. They contain various degrees of fats and glycerin, are less drying than acne soaps, and are not as creamy as super-fatted soaps.

Castile soaps, named for their origin in northern Spain, are prepared with olive oil. Olive oil is also a great moisturizer because it hydrates your skin without leaving a creamy residue.

Tone. Toners, often referred to as lotions or astringents, are used to remove debris remaining after cleansing. They also hydrate and reestablish the skin's proper pH. Toners come in alcohol-based and non-alcohol-based versions. Witch hazel is a great non-alcohol alternative. It cleans your skin like alcohol but isn't drying or irritating.

For normal to dry skin: Use a non-alcohol toner with a witch hazel, citrus, or essential oil base.

For oily or acne skin: Use a witch hazel–based formula. People with acne often prefer alcohol-based toners because it dries their blemishes and makes their skin feel clean. Alcohol, however, irritates the skin. Tea tree oil has the same antibacterial effect as alcohol without damaging your skin. Gently apply a drop of tea tree oil into your problem area(s), and massage. Repeat two or three times a day until your blemish is gone. Avoid eye contact.

Apply serum. The function of a serum is to give the deeper layers of your skin added nutrients, moisture, and protection. There are many types of serums, such as anti-aging, acne prevention, wrinkle reducing, and skin brightening. Serums generally come in liquid form and are applied after your toner and before your moisturizer.

Moisturize. Regular use of your favorite day and nighttime moisturizer is crucial.

Day creams seal in moisture to prevent water loss and add oil or control oil production. A good day cream will contain anti-inflammatory ingredients, such as aloe vera, balm mint, golden seaweed extract, or marine pine

9-1-1 RESCUE THERAPY: ACNE

Acne is one of the more common skin conditions I treat in my practice. It responds very well to acupuncture. Outbreaks can happen to anyone; here is a trick to help get rid of a blemish quickly:

Grind an aspirin into powder and add just enough water to form a paste. Apply it to the affected area and leave it on overnight. By morning the pimple should be gone or well on its way.

For stubborn cases of acne, use this acupressure regime, which is modeled after the acupuncture procedure I perform in my office. Do ten rotations of each point in a clockwise direction for a total of three times. Massage these points daily for at least twenty days and you should see noticeable results.

Stomach 36 | ST 36 is located on the outside of the leg below the knee in the depression approximately four fingers-widths below the outside of the leg bone, or fibula.

Spleen 10 | In a seated position with one knee bent, cup the palm of your hand around the bottom of the opposite knee. Slide your thumb to the inside of your knee. It should fall into a depression on the inside of the leg. This is SP 10.

Large Intestine 4 | Press your thumb to your index finger until it forms a crease on the back of your hand. This point is at the end of the crease.

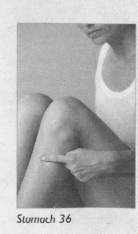

Stomach 36

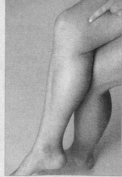

Spleen 10

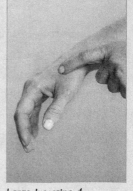

Large Intestine 4

Large Intestine 11 | Bend your elbow into your body at a 90-degree angle. LI 11 is at the elbow, on the outside edge of the elbow crease.

Lung 9 | Bend your wrist forward toward your arm. L 9 is located in the crease of your wrist, below your thumb, between the thumb bone and the tendon.

Triple Heater 17 | TH 17 is located in the depression below the ears at the base of the skull.

Stomach 3 | ST 3 is located directly below the center of your eye at the level of the nostrils.

Stomach 7 | ST 7 is located in front of your ear. You can find it by feeling for the depression between the cheekbone and the jawbone.

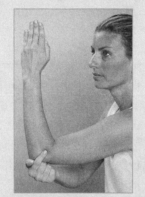

Large Intestine 11

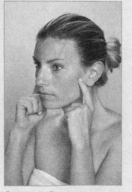

Lung 9

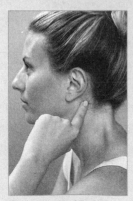

Triple Heater 17

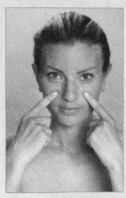

Stomach 3

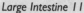

Stomach 7

bark to counteract the harmful effects of the sun's rays, pollution, and other environmental irritants.

Night creams correct skin problems. They are usually thicker than daytime moisturizers and target a specific skin condition. Make sure to get one that targets your skin type.

There is controversy regarding the use of night creams. Some people say that you should wear nothing on your skin at night so that it can breathe. However, nighttime is also the time when the body rests and repairs itself. A little help can go a long way, and night creams fit the bill. I highly recommend them. Some people also claim that day and night moisturizers are the same. Day and night creams that are designed to do their job are not the same, so I recommend separating them.

Use sunblock and sunscreen. Protecting your face from the sun is a must if you want to retain a youthful look. There are two ways to do it: use sunscreen or sunblock.

Sunblocks are opaque creams that physically block visible light and harmful sun rays. Zinc oxide is the most common natural ingredient found in sunblocks. There is another effective sunblock, titanium dioxide, but its safety is controversial.

Sunscreens are thinner in consistency and contain chemicals that protect your skin by absorbing and reflecting the harmful rays of the sun. Examples of ingredients found in sunscreens are zinc oxide and Parsol 1789, although the jury is still out on the safety of Parsol 1789. Natural sunscreens currently on the market use zinc oxide in combination with sun-damage-healing agents such as aloe vera, seaweed extract, sea buckthorn berry, and marine pine bark. Cocoa butter, vitamin E, and jojoba oil are also added to replenish skin moisture.

Weekly Essential

Write *you* into your calendar!

Put ten to fifteen minutes into your schedule once or twice a week to revitalize your skin, stimulate cell renewal, and focus your attention on a healthy and vibrant appearance for your face.

Exfoliate. As skin cells float to the surface of the epidermis and die, they need to be removed. Exfoliants are products that slough off dead cells from the surface of the skin. In addition, exfoliating helps remove dry, flaky patches and soften clogged pores. Exfoliating gives your skin a soft, smooth, fresh appearance. Exfoliants should be used after washing your face and before toning. When properly used, you can see and feel the difference. Exfoliants come in many forms.

Chemical exfoliants, commonly referred to as alpha hydroxy acids, dissolve surface skin buildup. They should be used with caution, as using them too much or too often can burn your skin. You will know when this happens because your skin will become irritated and red.

Enzyme exfoliants are the acids from the pulp of fruits, vegetables, or dairy products that digest dead surface cells. The most common come from pineapple, papaya, pumpkin, milk, yogurt, and kefir. They are gentler than chemical exfoliants and are easy to make yourself.

Gommage exfoliants take their name from the French word *gommage,* which means "to erase." Gommage exfoliants are generally gels that get tacky as they dry on the skin. As you rub them off, they lift and erase dead surface cells.

Exfoliant scrubs feel grainy and are made with substances such as ground nutshells, cornmeal, and sugar. Although effective, they can be abrasive and irritating, particularly to sensitive skin. Exfoliant scrubs that use oatmeal or rice powder are alternatives that are less harsh and easier on your skin.

Use a mask. Masks are the key to repairing your skin. A facial mask not only makes your skin look better, but also improves skin health. A facial mask is a thick lotion or paste that you put all over your face and leave on for a set amount of time, usually about twenty minutes. There are many types of masks. Some flush out accumulated toxins or clear up blemishes. Other masks repair, hydrate, or firm your skin. The short-term benefits of a good mask should be visible even after one application. Basic facial mask ingredients include oatmeal, honey, lemon juice, avocado, cucumber, yogurt, and milk.

How to Read a Label: It's More Than Skin Deep

Controversy looms in the skin care industry, meaning you should choose your products carefully. Deciding which ingredients to use and which to avoid is essential to your health and well-being. More and more companies are altering their formulas to become safer and environmentally friendly.

Mainstream skin care companies and all-natural or organic skin care lines differ in their views of what is safe and what is not only unsafe but harmful to your skin. Health advocates point out that much of the controversy stems from independent studies that focus on using high-dose levels of toxic substances rather than the effects of chronic low-level damage caused by applying these ingredients to your skin day after day. In addition, many of the larger, well-known companies believe that the biological effects of most chemicals are the same whether they are isolated from natural sources or synthesized in a lab.

Proponents of all-natural skin care believe that natural substances are safer and more effective than their synthetic counterparts. Organic ingredients are cultivated without the use of harmful pesticides and are preferred by many health-conscious skin care companies. Ultimately the choice is yours; however, here is what you should know about the most controversial ingredients commonly found in many skin care products.

Glycols. Polyethylene glycol (PEG) and propylene glycol (PPG) have similar properties and are added to skin care products to improve their ability to penetrate into your skin. They are also used in antifreeze, airplane de-icers, brake fluid, paint, and floor shampoos. According to the safety data sheets of industrial chemical manufacturers, PPG and PEG can be irritants to the eyes, skin, and mucous membranes. Although research shows that PEGs are less harmful than PPGs, both are a source of controversy. Glycerol is now substituted as a natural alternative to PEG and PPG.

Parabens. For years, parabens (butyl, ethyl, methyl, and propyl) have been used as synthetic preservatives in skin and beauty care products, such as face creams, shampoos, conditioners, and deodorants. Since 1988, reports have claimed that parabens mimic the female hormone estrogen, and the use of them may be linked to cancer and birth defects. Although controversy still exists, there is enough compelling evidence to spur a rapidly growing trend in paraben-free products. Healthy substitutes for parabens include grapefruit seed extract, vitamin E, and oils such as cinnamon, eucalyptus, lavender, tea tree, and lemon.

Sodium lauryl sulfate / sodium laureth sulfate. Sodium lauryl sulfate (SLS) and sodium laureth sulfate (SLES) are used as lathering agents in skin care products. They are also used in floor cleaners and car wash detergents and to melt grease in car engines. On your skin, they dissolve healthy oils and can make your skin very dry. An alternative to SLS and SLES is glycyrrhizin, which is a natural derivative of licorice root.

Synthetic colors and dyes. On labels, you'll see the letters FD&C and D&C followed by a color and a number (for instance, FD&C Red No. 4 and D&C Green No. 6). They are generally derived from coal tar,

---

SKIN ALLERGY PATCH TEST

In order to determine whether a product or skin care recipe is right for you, it is important to conduct a skin allergy patch test. Here are the instructions.

- Clean a quarter-size area of skin on either your neck or the inside of your wrist.
- With a clean cotton ball or Q-tip, apply the product or skin care recipe to the cleaned test spot.
- Let the test spot dry. Do not wash or cover for twenty-four hours.
- Examine the area periodically over the twenty-four-hour period. If you experience any redness, burning, itching, swelling, skin abrasion, eruption, or irritation in or around the test spot, do not use the product without consulting your doctor first.

chromium oxide, or aluminum powder, and according to the Material Safety Data Sheet, they range from mild irritants to potential carcinogens. Natural vegetable dyes can be substituted as a healthy alternative.

Choosing Your Products

My favorite skin care products contain natural and organic ingredients. I have tried hundreds of products over the years, and my favorites always seem to be those containing natural ingredients. My barometer? The results they achieve.

When shopping for natural products, look for those that not only carry the organic seal but are eco-certified as well. This means that the manufacturing and packaging plants have also undergone rigorous testing and uphold the highest integrity.

These are the product lines I use and recommend to my patients. You can find out more about them and how to purchase them by going to my website, at www.hamptonsacupuncture.com.

AUBREY ORGANICS

Aubrey Organics was one of the first organic skin care products on the market and is still going strong. With more than forty years of experience, this product line's claim to fame is its use of hand-grown and -harvested aloe vera as a base ingredient.

ÉMINENCE ORGANIC SKIN CARE OF HUNGARY

An award-winning provider of skin care products, Éminence uses sustainable farming and green practices to create handmade organic products. You can actually see the seeds, pulp, and peel in their formulas.

KIEHL'S

Founded in New York in 1851, this authentic apothecary, which is still located in New York City, carries an extensive blend of face and body cosmetics. Its açaí skin care line is organic and free of parabens and other harmful ingredients.

LABORATORIES LUZERN

Luzern's skin care ingredients are cultivated at high altitudes in the Swiss Alps. This organic paraben- and preservative-free line uses pharmaceutical-grade ingredients for immediate and long-lasting results.

NATUROPATHICA

The company motto is "a better beauty," and the products truly live up to it. This aromatherapy-based line is both organic and eco-certified. I frequently recommend it to my patients.

NEAL'S YARD REMEDIES

Neal's Yard Remedies started in 1981 in Neal's Yard Covent Garden, in the heart of central London. It is claimed to be the first certified organic health and beauty company in the United Kingdom, and still offers the largest range of certified organic health and beauty products.

NEFELI

Nefeli products are designed by Ping Zhang, a fourth-generation Chinese herbalist and practitioner of Traditional Chinese medicine. The formulas and ingredients are based on the principles of Chinese medicine.

THE ORGANIC PHARMACY

Established by pharmacist Margo Marrone, this British-based company offers a skin care line that is all-organic and environmentally friendly, and that uses no animal testing, artificial preservatives, mineral oils, paraffins, synthetic chemicals, or artificial fragrances or colors.

ORIGINS

Founded in 1990, Origins has grown to become one of the largest retail, natural, and certified organic product industries. Origins stores are located countrywide. The company logo is "Powered by nature, proven by science," and it has teamed up with well-known natural physician and skin care expert Dr. Andrew Weil in order to help live up to it. Origins skin care ingredients are 100 percent natural and formulated without parabens, phthalates, polypropylene glycol, mineral oil, PABA, petrolatum, paraffins, or animal ingredients.

RADICAL SKINCARE

Radical Skincare is a new line of products developed in California by sisters Rachel and Elizabeth Edlich. Their products use resveratrol and other high-potency, peptide-infused antioxidants from berries, grapeseed extract, green tea, and coffeeberry. Although the ingredients are not 100 percent organic, they are radical!

WELEDA

With more than ninety years of skin care experience, Weleda is one of the world's original organic skin care lines. Ingredients are cultivated in the company's own biodynamic gardens.

YON-KA PARIS

Created by two botanists in France, Yon-Ka merges four therapies (aroma, plant, marine, and fruit acid) into an extensive line of nurturing, therapeutic, and healing products. Although the products are not 100 percent natural, they are holistically formulated, extremely effective, and worth every ounce.

12

The Perfect Match: Finding the Right Practitioner for You

NOW THAT YOU'VE READ THIS FAR, YOU MIGHT be thinking that working directly with an acupuncturist would benefit you. An acupuncturist can help you determine your Chinese Organ type and, with a few sessions of acupuncture, give you a jump start in using the programs in this book.

There are many highly qualified acupuncturists in the United States. Today there are more than 45,000 licensed acupuncturists in the country, compared with 20,000 five years ago, and more than 5,000 physician acupuncturists, compared with 1,800 five years ago. You have a lot of choices.

The relationship between you and your acupuncturist is a personal one. Like finding the right mate, finding the right acupuncturist depends on good vibes, communication, and trust. Following is information about acupuncture licensure and the steps you should take to find the right acupuncturist for you. If you already see an acupuncturist, or know someone who can recommend one, then you are ahead of the game.

STATE CERTIFICATION REQUIREMENTS

As of publication of this book, the following states allow only medical doctors, osteopaths, or chiropractors to practice acupuncture:

Alabama	Mississippi
Delaware	North Dakota
Kansas	Oklahoma
Minnesota	South Dakota

In these states, a licensed acupuncturist can practice under the supervision of a medical doctor or osteopath:

Kansas	Michigan
Louisiana	

In these states, you must obtain a referral from an M.D. in order to see an acupuncturist:

Nebraska	Ohio

These states require an acupuncturist to be licensed but do not require continuing education:

Colorado	Oregon
Connecticut	Pennsylvania
Georgia	Utah
Hawaii	Washington
Montana	Washington, D.C.
New York	Wisconsin

These states require an acupuncturist to be licensed and to submit proof of current active NCCAOM* certification in acupuncture as their only continuing education requirement:

Indiana	New Mexico
Kentucky	Ohio
Minnesota	South Carolina
Missouri	Tennessee
Nebraska	Virginia
New Hampshire	

The following states have their own requirements for licensure and continuing education:

Alaska	Maryland
Arizona	Massachusetts
Arkansas	New Jersey
California	Nevada
Florida	North Carolina
Illinois	Rhode Island
Indiana	Texas
Iowa	Vermont
Maine	West Virginia

*The National Certification Commission for Acupuncture and Oriental Medicine (NCCAOM).

Each state independently regulates the practice of medicine, whether it is allopathic (Western) or acupuncture (Eastern). Some states have strict acupuncture legislation and licensing requirements, while other states have no regulations at all. In order to enroll in acupuncture school in New York, for example, you must have sixty semester hours of undergraduate training, plus nine semester hours of bioscience. In order to graduate from an acupuncture program, you must complete 4,050 hours (equivalent to a three-year program) of training from an accredited acupuncture school. You must then successfully pass a written and practical exam and take a clean-needle-technique course. There are a few exceptions to this rule. Licensed physicians, osteopaths, and dentists with three hundred hours of acceptable training in acupuncture are referred to as certified acupuncturists and can legally practice acupuncture.

For further information, contact the American Academy of Medical Acupuncture (AAMA; www.medicalacupuncture.org). Auricular or ear acupuncture for the treatment of chemical dependency in a hospital or authorized treatment clinic can be performed by an acupuncture detoxification therapist (ADT) who has completed seventy hours of acupuncture training (thirty classroom hours, plus forty hours of hands-on clinical experience). The scope of practice for an ADT is limited to the insertion of a maximum of five points in each ear, and ADTs can perform this service only in their workplace under the supervision of a licensed or certified acupuncturist. You can learn more about this from the National Acupuncture Detoxification Association (NADA; www.acudetox.com).

In order to understand your local guidelines, contact the appropriate state governing body (usually the Department of State or the State Education Department). If you are computer-savvy, you can download guidelines on the Internet. For a free state-by-state listing, go to www.acufinder.com/Acupuncture+Laws.

The National Acupuncture Foundation publishes a handbook titled *Acupuncture and Oriental Medicine State Laws and Regulations* by Tierney Tully (2005 edition), which outlines the acupuncture requirements for each state. It is available for purchase through amazon.com.

The National Certification Commission for Acupuncture and Oriental Medicine (NCCAOM) is a private, nonprofit organization that develops, promotes, and administers examinations and certification for acupuncture and professions related to Chinese medicine. The NCCAOM upholds the standard of practice among acupuncturists nationwide. It was created to establish, assess, and promote recognized standards of competence and safety in acupuncture and Chinese medicine. Although its certification is not required by all states, many rely on this organization to provide and maintain acupuncture-related continuing education requirements, known as Professional Development Activity (PDA) points. For further information, go to www.nccaom.org or call 904-598-1005. State licensing guidelines and states that use the NCCAOM PDA system for maintaining licensure are detailed on page 224.

You can also contact the National Center for Complementary and Alternative Medicine (NCCAM). It has developed a fact sheet to provide you with information on acupuncture, http://nccam.nih.gov/health/acupuncture, which includes frequently asked questions, issues to consider, and a list of sources for further information.

For detailed information about acupuncture, acupuncture studies, or conditions that acupuncture treats, log on to the following websites:

www.nccam.nih.gov
www.AcuFinder.com
www.acupuncture.com

Questions to Ask

Once you have done your homework, located a potential acupuncturist, and are ready to make the call, here are a few questions that you can ask:

What are your specific credentials?

How long have you been in practice?

Do you use disposable sterile needles?

Have you ever treated someone with my condition?

What is your success rate with my condition?

Is there someone that you have treated with my condition whom I can contact? (In accordance with HIPA regulations, acupuncturists may or may not be able to divulge this information.)

How many appointments might someone with my condition typically need?

How much do you charge per visit? (Some practitioners may offer discounts for packages of treatments, or have a payment plan or a sliding scale.)

Are there additional fees that might be incurred (tests, supplements, equipment, etc.)?

Do you accept my health insurance?

If so, do I file the claim or do you?

If you feel comfortable with your conversation, then make an appointment.

In the first visit, you probably will be asked a number of questions. Here are a few things that your acupuncturist may want to know about you:

- Health history
- Medications (you may want to bring in a list)
- Diet
- Sleep
- Digestion
- Stress level
- Lifestyle
- Skin care regime (for cosmetic acupuncture)

Your practitioner will feel your wrist to take your pulse. As with the beat of your heart in Western medicine, in Chinese medicine you can feel the quality of your Organs in your wrist pulse. You will then be asked to stick out your tongue. This may sound like a strange request, but again it helps your acupuncturist assess your internal condition. You then may be asked to lie down so the acupuncturist can press a few of your acupuncture points.

Now the fun begins. After explaining the findings and answering your questions, your acupuncturist will begin inserting fine, sterile acupuncture needles into strategic points, according to your individual condition. You may feel an initial pinch while the needle is being inserted, but once it is in place, you should have no discomfort. If a point bothers you, simply ask your acupuncturist to adjust the needle.

Although no two people have the same experience, some report feelings of something (Qi?) flowing through their body. Many people fall asleep, while others report a sensation of floating in and out of a semi dream state. Even better, after repeat treatments, you will begin to notice something different. Stressful situations no longer seem intolerable, life is calmer, and you start to feel both energetic and relaxed. This is balance, and what you are experiencing is your body thanking you for helping to find its long-lost state of well-being.

Appendix
Key Acupressure Points

FOOT

Liver 2 (LV 2)

This point is located on top of the foot between your first and second toes.
It is used cosmetically to:

- Reduce wrinkles between the eyebrows and around the eyes
- Reduce redness and irritation in the eyes

Massaging the point can also help ease these conditions:

- Dizziness
- Eczema
- Headache
- Migraine (lateral)
- Rosacea (some forms)

Liver 3 (LV 3)

This point is located on the top of your foot, one finger-width behind LV 2. Slide your finger between these two toes toward the top of your foot. When you reach the intersection of the first and second toe, you are on the spot. It is the primary point for smoothing the Liver Qi. It is used to treat:

- Wrinkles
- Sunspots
- Muscle spasms
- Headache
- Vision problems
- Stress
- Pain

Gallbladder 43 (GB 43)

This point is located in the web between your fourth and last (little) toe. It is used to reduce Liver heat and Liver fire. It is used to:

- Diminish wrinkles on the forehead
- Clear eye redness
- Calm the mind
- Treat one-sided (temporal) headaches

Spleen 3 (SP 3)

This point is located on the inside of your foot, below the head of the large toe, on the edge of the dark and light skin. This is the primary point for strengthening weak Spleen Qi and eliminating Spleen dampness. It is used to treat:

- Sagging muscles
- Allergies
- Cellulite
- Edema
- Digestive problems
- Sinusitis

Kidney 3 (K 3)

This point is located in the soft spot on the inside of your ankle, between the inside ankle bone and the tendon. This is the primary point for strengthening weak Kidney Yin, Yang, and Essence. It can also be used to help deter:

- Premature aging
- Hair loss
- Dark undereye circles
- Eye or facial puffiness
- Fatigue

Kidney 6 (K 6)

This point is located on the inside of your foot, directly below the ankle bone. This point is used to nourish Kidney Yin, moisten dryness, and cool the Blood. It is also used for these conditions:

- Dry lips
- Hair thinning
- Ringing in the ears

LEG

Spleen 6 (SP 6)

This point is located on the inside of the leg, roughly four finger-widths above the top of the ankle (medial) bone. It is at the intersection of the Yin leg Meridians of the Liver, Kidneys, and Spleen. It balances and strengthens the Qi and Blood of these Organs and is good for lifting facial and body muscles. It is also used for treating:

- Allergies
- Skin problems
- Digestive disorders
- Weight gain

Bladder 60 (BL 60)

This point is located in the back of the leg, behind the knee. It is used to relax the neck, head, and face. It is also used for treating:

- Neck pain
- Back pain
- Headaches
- Painful menstrual periods

Stomach 36 (ST 36)

This point is located in the depression four finger-widths below the bottom of your knee, on the outside of the leg bone (fibula). This point lifts cheek muscles, strengthens the digestive system, and improves immune function. It can also be used to strengthen the immune system.

Gallbladder 34 (GB 34)

This point is located below the outside of the knee, at the head of the fibula (the outside of the leg bone). This point is used to clear heat from the Gallbladder and Liver. It smooths Liver Qi and is therefore used to relax muscles, soften wrinkles, and resolve any condition that involves a Liver Qi imbalance. It can also be used for:

- Headache (lateral)

Bladder 40 (BL 40)

This point is located in the back of the knee between the two tendons. It is used to:

- Reduce redness and irritation in the face and body
- Alleviate back pain

Spleen 10 (SP 10)

This point is located three finger-widths above the inside of your knee. In a seated position with your knee bent, cup the palm of your hand around the bottom of the opposite knee. Slide your thumb upward to the inside of your knee. It should fall into a depression on the inside of the leg. This point is used to:

- Stimulate blood circulation
- Reduce redness and irritation
- Restore rosy cheeks
- Minimize sunspots

It is also is used to treat these conditions:

- Acne
- Blemishes
- Eczema

- Eye irritation
- Rosacea

HAND

Large Intestine 4 (LI 4)

Press your thumb to your index finger until it forms a crease on the back of your hand. This point is at the end of the crease. Pressing this point sends Qi to your face. It is the main point for eliminating wind-heat. It is used cosmetically to:

- Reduce redness
- Clear irritated skin
- Lift and tone facial muscles

In addition, it can be used to treat these conditions:

- Colds and flu
- Eye irritation
- Headache
- Nasal congestion
- Sinusitis

Lung 9 (L 9)

Bend your wrist forward toward your arm. This point is located in the crease of your wrist, below your thumb, between the thumb bone and the tendon. This is the primary point for strengthening Lung Qi and Lung Yin. It is used to:

- Moisten dry skin
- Reduce puffiness and congestion in the face
- Balance pore size

Heart 7 (HT 7)

This point is located on the inside wrist at the crease where the wrist bends, on the spot between the tendons in line with the little finger. This is the primary point for balancing the Heart. It is used to:

- Reduce redness
- Improve circulation in the face
- Relax the spirit

ARM

Lung 7 (L 7)

This point is located on the lower portion of the arm, one finger-width above L 9, on the inside of the thumb bone. It is used to get rid of wind-cold and wind-heat. It is used to treat:

- Acne
- Allergies
- Blemishes
- Colds
- Coughs
- Nasal congestion
- Sinusitis
- Sinus-related headaches

Pericardium 6 (P 6)

This point is located on the inside of the arm, between the two tendons, three finger-widths from the crease of the wrist. This balances Blood flow in the face, protecting and calming the Heart.

Large Intestine 11 (LI 11)

Bend your elbow into your body at a 90-degree angle. This point is at the elbow, on the outside edge of the elbow crease. This point is often used with LI 4 to get rid of wind-heat. It sends Qi to the face. It is used cosmetically to:

- Tone muscles
- Eliminate redness, including that associated with acne
- Reduce puffiness
- Get rid of blemishes

It also helps clear:

- Nasal and sinus congestion

NECK

Governing Vessel 14 (GV 14)

If you slide your fingers from the top of your shoulder to the top of your spine, you will find this point. It is located on top of the spine, between the seventh cervical and first thoracic vertebrae. As the meeting point of all Yang Meridians, this point has many functions. It brings Yang Qi to the head, strengthens the Heart Qi, and clears wind-heat.

It is also used to:

- Clear the mind and stimulate the brain
- Lift and tone facial muscles
- Reduce facial puffiness
- Diminish sunspots
- Brighten the face
- Treat colds, flu, sinusitis, and nasal congestion

Bladder 10 (BL 10)

Place your fingers in the center of your spine, below the base of your skull. Slide your hand toward your ear until you land in a notch approximately one finger-width away. This point opens the back of the neck to increase the flow of Qi and Blood to the head. It can therefore be used with any facial acupressure treatment. It helps relieve Kidney/Bladder headaches in the back of the neck and on the top and front of the head. It has a special effect on the eyes and can improve vision in cases of Kidney deficiency. It also gets rid of wind-cold and wind-heat in the head and is effective for these conditions:

- Colds and flu
- Nasal congestion
- Sinusitis

Gallbladder 20 (GB 20)

From BL 10, slide your hands another finger-width away from the center of the spine. This point opens the back of the neck to increase the flow of Qi and Blood to the head. Like BL 10, this point has many functions. It helps relieve Liver/Gallbladder headaches in the back and on the side of the head. It has a significant effect on the eyes. It relaxes muscle tension and wrinkles around the eyes, improves vision in cases of Liver Yin deficiency, and reduces eye redness from Liver Yang and fire excess. It also eliminates wind-cold and wind-heat and can be used to treat these conditions:

- Colds and flu
- Dizziness

- Nasal congestion
- Sinusitis

Triple Heater 17 (TH 17)

This point is located in the depression below the ears at the base of the skull. It is the primary lymphatic drainage point for the face. It is used cosmetically to:

- Reduce congestion, swelling, and puffiness in the face

It is also the major point for treating:

- Ear problems

Small Intestine 17 (SI 17)

From Triple Heater (TH) 17, slide your fingers in front of the SCM muscle (the long muscle extending from the jaw to the collarbone). This is Small Intestine 17. This point is used to:

- Relax tight neck muscles
- Tighten loose skin in the neck
- Assist in lymph drainage

Conception Vessel 23 (CV 23)

This point is located on your neck, above the Adam's apple, directly below the center of the chin. This point connects the muscles of the neck with the muscle of the chin. It is used to:

- Lift the muscles of the neck and chin

FACE

Conception Vessel 24 (CV 24)

This point is located in the center of your chin, below the middle of the lower lip. This point is used to:

- Lift all the muscles of the face, particularly those around the mouth and neck
- Reduce facial swelling and puffiness

It is effective for treating:

- Bell's palsy
- Facial paralysis

Governing Vessel 26 (GV 26)
This point is located in the soft tissue below the tip of your nose and above the center of your upper lip. It is used to:

- Increase circulation to the face and head
- Improve a pale or puffy complexion

It is also used to treat:

- Back pain

Large Intestine 19 (LI 19)
This point is located below your nostril and above your upper lip. It is used to:

- Reduce wrinkles above your lips

Large Intestine 20 (LI 20)
This point is located on the sides of your nostrils. It is used to:

- Lift and tone sagging cheek muscles

With ST 3, it also relieves:

- Nasal and sinus congestion

Stomach 2 (ST 2)
This point is located at the center of the eye directly below the eye bone. It is used to:

- Lift and tone sagging cheek muscles
- Reduce eye redness
- Soften wrinkles around the eyes

Stomach 3 (ST 3)
This point is located directly below the center of the eye at the level of the nostrils. It is used to:

- Lift and tone sagging cheek muscles

With LI 20, it is also used to relieve:

- Nasal and sinus congestion

Stomach 4 (ST 4)

This point is located directly below ST 3, at the corner of the mouth. It is used to:

- Lift and tone sagging cheek muscles

Stomach 5 (ST 5)

This point is located above the jawline, one finger-width in front of ST 6. With ST 4 and ST 6 it:

- Relaxes the jaw and tightens sagging jawlines

Stomach 6 (ST 6)

This point is located on your cheek, one finger-width above the angle of the jaw. It is used to:

- Lift and tone cheek muscles and tighten sagging jawlines

Stomach 7 (ST 7)

This point is located in front of your ear. You can find it by feeling for the depression between the cheekbone and the jawbone. It is used to:

- Lift and tone cheek muscles

Stomach 8 (ST 8)

This point is located at the edge of the forehead at the bend in your hairline. It is used to:

- Lift and tone muscles of the cheek and forehead

It is also used to relieve:

- Frontal and temporal headaches

Small Intestine 18 (SI 18)

This point is located on the cheek, directly below the outer edge of the eye and to the side of the nose. It is used to:

- Lift and tone cheek muscles
- Lift the corners of the mouth

It is also used to treat:
- Bell's palsy
- Facial paralysis

Bladder 1 (BL 1)
This point is located in the inner corner of the eyes. It is used for:
- All eye problems

Bladder 2 (BL 2)
This point is located at the inside edge of the eyebrows, above the inside corner of the eye. It is used to:
- Release tension in the face and forehead
- Reduce creases between the eyebrows and forehead
- Relax the mind

Bladder 3 (BL 3)
This point is located in the hairline directly above BL 2. Move your fingers straight up your forehead to the base of the hairline. This is BL 3. It is used to:
- Relax forehead wrinkles

Yu Yao
This is an extra point, meaning it's not on an Organ Meridian. It is located in the middle of the eyebrow. It is used to:
- Soften wrinkles between the eyebrow and across the forehead

It is also used to treat:
- Tension and pain around the eyes
- Blurred vision or floaters

Gallbladder 1 (GB 1)
This point is located at the outside corner of the eyes. It is effective for many eye problems, among them:
- Relaxing eye strain
- Reducing redness
- Treating wrinkles around the eyes

Gallbladder 13 (GB 13)

Divide your hairline as if you had a center part. Follow your hairline from the front center to approximately three finger-widths across the hairline. This is GB 13. This point is used for:

- Wrinkles on the forehead

Gallbladder 14 (GB 14)

This point is located on your forehead, one finger-width above the center of the eyebrows. This is a primary point for:

- Wrinkles on the forehead and between the eyebrows

It is also used to treat:

- Headache
- Facial paralysis

Gallbladder 15 (GB 15)

This point is located directly above GB 14 in the hairline. This is a primary point for:

- Wrinkles on the forehead

It is also used to treat:

- Headache

Yin Tang

This point is located between the eyebrows and above the nose. It relaxes the face and body, and clears the head. It is used to:

- Reduce creases between the eyebrows
- Induce relaxation

Governing Vessel 20 (GV 20)

This point is located on the top of the head. You can locate it by placing your thumbs on the top of your ears and your finger on the top of your head. The point is where your fingers meet. It is used to:

- Improve circulation in the face
- Lift sagging face muscles
- Clear and calm the mind

Glossary

These are common terms used in this book as they pertain to Chinese medicine.

Acne   Inflammation of the skin from underlying oil or debris.

AcuFacial®   The author's signature treatment to firm loose facial muscles, eliminate fine lines, soften deep wrinkles, and improve overall skin tone. It combines acupuncture, ultrasound, light-emitting diode (LED), anti-aging creams, and dietary recommendations.

AcuFacial® Acupressure Facelift   The author's signature do-it-yourself program, modeled after AcuFacial®, that firms loose facial muscles, eliminates fine lines, softens deep wrinkles, and improves overall skin tone.

Acupressure   An ancient Chinese healing method that employs manual massage on acupuncture points on the body to relieve symptoms and treat body imbalances. It is used to treat illnesses and, cosmetically, to address aging.

Acupressure/acupuncture point   A precise point on the body that, when stimulated, helps balance the body and mind. There are more than 365 points in the body. This book uses forty-six of them to address the visible signs of aging.

Acupuncture   An ancient Chinese healing method that involves the insertion of fine needles into specific points on the body to relieve symptoms and treat body imbalances.

Acupuncture needles   Thin, sterile stainless-steel needles that are inserted into specific sites on the body for the purpose of obtaining a desired effect.

Alopecia   Hair loss leading to patches of baldness.

Allergy   A sensitivity to foods, chemicals, or foreign substances that causes an internal or external heightened immune reaction.

Alternative medicine   The use of nontraditional Western medicine for the purpose of promoting health and well-being.

Anti-wrinkle cream   A commercial or homemade skin care product containing antioxidants and other skin-enhancing compounds designed to reduce the appearance of deep wrinkles and eliminate fine wrinkles.

Bacteria   Microbes or germs that exist in multiple strains.

Blood   In Chinese medicine, Blood is a Yin substance that travels through the body with Qi to moisten and nourish the body. It is produced, stored, and circulated throughout the Organs and Meridians.

Blood deficiency   A lack of Blood moving through the Organs and Meridians that can cause a weakness or weaknesses in one or more Organs.

Blood stagnation   A condition in which Blood becomes sluggish or stops moving.

Botox   The commercial name for botulinum. It is injected into the muscle to soften or inhibit the formation of wrinkles. It works by temporarily blocking muscle receptors that cause muscles to contract.

Capillaries   Small blood vessels that connect arteries to veins.

Cells The "building blocks" of the body, according to Western medicine. Each cell contains all of the information necessary for the physical existence of each individual.

Chinese medicine An ancient and complex healing system, practiced in the Eastern world, that is seeded in the prevention of disease. Treatment is addressed through establishing optimum movement of Qi through twelve Organ systems in the body.

Circulation In Chinese medicine, it is the passage of Qi and/or Blood throughout the body's Organ system.

Cleanser A face-washing substance and the first step in a daily skin care regimen.

Cold One of Chinese medicine's six evils, characterized by feeling chilled or cold and an intolerance for cold weather conditions. It is associated with the Kidney Organ system.

Collagen A substance that forms the underlying support and resilience of skin.

Complementary and alternative medicine (CAM) A term used to describe medical practices and beliefs that fall outside of Western medical beliefs and practices.

Conception Vessel One of the body's extra Meridian networks. It governs the Yin aspect and Yin Organ systems of the body.

Dampness One of Chinese medicine's six evils, characterized by a feeling of heaviness or sluggishness. It can be associated with copious discharge of fluids or an inability to lose weight. Dampness is often accompanied by heat or cold. It is generally associated with the Spleen Organ system.

Day cream A product applied to the face and worn throughout the day.

Deficiency The underactivity or lacking of a particular substance in the body.

Dehydration A lack of water and other life-sustaining fluids in the body.

Dermis The middle layer of skin located between the epidermis and hypodermis.

Dryness One of Chinese medicine's six evils, characterized by the feeling of thirst and dehydration. It is associated with the Lung Organ system.

Eastern medicine See *Chinese medicine.*

Eczema An inflammatory skin condition characterized by redness, irritation, and itching.

Edema An abnormal accumulation of fluid or swelling under the surface of the skin.

Elastin This substance, located in the dermal layer of the skin, provides skin elasticity and prevents skin looseness.

Epidermis The outermost layer of the skin.

Essence The embodiment of Qi and Blood that we cannot live without. It encompasses an individual's existence—physically, mentally, emotionally, and spiritually. Essence is both Yin and Yang.

Essential oils Highly concentrated extracts from plants used for healing and cosmetic purposes.

Esthetician A specialist in skin care health and beauty.

Esthetics A philosophy pertaining to skin care forms of beauty.

Excess Too much of a particular substance or a condition of overactivity.

Exfoliate The removal of excessive debris from the surface of the skin.

Face mask A skin care product applied to the face.

Fire One of Chinese medicine's six evils, characterized by extreme dryness, heat, or fever. Fire is associated with the Heart Organ system.

Flavor A description of a food as either one or a combination of bitter, salty, sour, spicy, or sweet.

Free radicals In Western medicine, these are damaged "renegade" cells that break away from healthy cells and create disease and cause premature aging.

Genetics The general term for the characteristics inherited from one's ancestors.

Glabellar crease The medical term for the fold or wrinkle between the eyebrows.

Governing Vessel   One of Chinese medicine's extra Meridian networks. It controls the Yang aspect and Yang Organ systems of the body.

Heart   One of Chinese medicine's Yin Organ systems. Known as the king of emotions, the Heart takes Qi essence from the Spleen and, with the Kidneys, makes and transports Blood throughout the Organ and Meridian systems. It affects skin coloring and complexion.

Heat   A pattern of disharmony characterized by a feeling of warmth, intolerance for cold, red complexion, and irritated skin. Also associated with one of the six evils.

Hydration   Pertaining to the maintenance of moisture in the body.

Immune system   In Western medicine, it governs the body's ability to resist disease.

Integrative medicine   The integration of Western and alternative medicine in a therapeutic setting.

Kidneys   One of Chinese medicine's Yin Organ systems. Known as the Root of Life, the Kidneys store essence and Qi. They are responsible for appropriate aging and the proper functioning of all of the Organ and Meridian systems.

Large Intestine   One of Chinese medicine's Yang Organ systems. It processes solid matter and keeps skin moist and healthy. It is paired with the Lungs.

Liver   One of Chinese medicine's Yin Organ systems. It governs the smooth flow of Qi throughout the body, stores and regulates Blood volume, and maintains healthy tendons, vision, and nails. It is the primary Organ system for treating wrinkles.

Lungs   One of Chinese medicine's Yin Organ systems. The Lungs transform and distribute air throughout the body and oversee the moisture content in the skin and body and the texture and general condition of the skin and body hair. The Lungs, through the production of protective Qi, also help maintain a healthy immune system.

Lymphatic system   A network of lymph vessels, lacteals, and nodes through which lymph flows throughout the body.

Meridians   Invisible pathways or channels through which Qi and Blood travel. Most acupuncture points are located on Meridians. There are fourteen Meridians.

Nasolabial fold   The medical term for the crease between the sides of the nose and corners of the mouth.

Night cream   A product applied to the face that is worn throughout the night.

Nourishing cycle   A structure through which one Organ system feeds or nourishes another.

Oil gland   An opening in the skin through which greasy liquids are released.

Oxidation   A process recognized by Western medicine in which a combination of oxygen and other toxic and foreign substances age and damage cells.

Oxygen   A gaseous substance necessary for plant, animal, and human existence.

Pericardium   One of Chinese medicine's Yin Organ systems. The Pericardium is associated with the Heart and Blood circulation.

Phlegm   A type of congestion caused by a concentration of the Chinese evil dampness. Although primarily associated with the Spleen, phlegm can accumulate anywhere in the body and is associated with the inability to lose weight.

Qi   Yang substance known in Chinese medicine as "vital energy." It is an invisible force that is the root of all life forms. Within the body it is produced, stored, and circulated throughout the Organ and Meridian systems.

Rosacea   Blotchy redness in the face characterized by flushing, breakouts, redness, and spider veins. It is sometimes referred to as adult acne.

Serum   A highly concentrated lotion containing anti-aging compounds designed to reduce wrinkles, eliminate fine lines, and tone and strengthen facial and neck skin.

Shen   A form of Essence or true being that encompasses consciousness, the mind, and all higher spiritual connections.

Sinusitis   Pertaining to congestion and inflammation in the sinus areas.

Six evils   External influences that, in Chinese medicine, cause illness. They are cold, dampness, dryness, heat/fire, summer heat, and wind.

Skin condition   The quality of the skin, especially the face, as it is affected by diet, the environment, and skin care maintenance.

Skin type   The quality of skin that Western medicine says is inherited and often determined by one's lineage and ethnicity. There are five skin types. Chinese medicine believes there is only one skin type—normal. Oiliness, dryness, and so on are signs of an Organ imbalance.

Small Intestine   One of Chinese medicine's Yang Organ systems. It assists in sending unwanted matter to the Organs of elimination. It is paired with the Heart.

Stagnation   Insufficient, blocked, or improper circulation of Qi and/or Blood.

Stomach   One of Chinese medicine's Yang Organ systems. Paired with the Spleen, it receives matter from the Spleen to be processed and digested.

Subcutaneous layer   The deepest layer of the skin. In Chinese medicine, muscles are also included in this layer.

Sunspots   Flat, brown spots of discoloration in the skin, commonly found on the hands, face, arms, and shoulders. They are also called liver spots.

Sweat glands   Openings in the skin through which fluid is excreted.

Toner   A skin refresher and soother, often referred to as lotion, used after washing the face.

Tonify   To strengthen weaknesses in Organs.

Tongue diagnosis   A Chinese medicine form of examination characterized by looking at the size, shape, texture, coating, and color of the tongue, used to make a diagnosis.

Triple Heater   One of Chinese medicine's Yang Organ systems. It is paired with the Pericardium and balances the upper, middle, and lower aspects of the body. It is also used to regulate the interior and exterior layers of skin, muscles, Organs, and Meridians.

Tui Na   Specific type of Chinese acupressure and the type the acupressure massages in this book are modeled after.

Ultraviolet (UV) radiation.   Invisible rays of the spectrum, which, when emitted by the sun, are most damaging to skin.

Western medicine   A complex system of health care practiced in the Western world that includes invasive techniques and pharmaceuticals to treat disease.

Wind   One of Chinese medicine's six evils. It causes muscle spasms, twitching, and pain and is associated with the Liver Organ system.

Wrinkle   A small ridge or furrow in the facial skin. In Western medicine, wrinkles are considered a natural part of aging. In Chinese medicine, they are associated with an imbalance in the Organ systems.

Yang   One of the two opposing forces of energy characterized by light, heat, and activity.

Yin   One the two opposing forces of energy characterized by dark, cold, and tranquility.

Yin Tang   An acupuncture/acupressure point located between the eyebrows and part of the AcuFacial® Acupressure Facelift. This point is called an extra point, as it is not found on a specific Meridian.

Acknowledgments

I would like to thank and dedicate this book to Colette Roy, for standing by my side with unending support, understanding, and delicious recipes; and to my parents, Alan and Vivian; my sisters Lisa and Cathy; and Neil, Dianne, Kevin, Jason, and the Golden/Gutman/Roy clans, because you are my family and you each mean the world to me.

I am grateful to my friends who care about me, believe in me, and cheer me on. Alice and Karen, thank you for your words of literary wisdom at all hours of the New York days and California nights.

Thank you to Diane Kraus, Elise D'Haene, and Stacey Donovan for getting me started. To Debora Yost, my editor, and Carol Mann, my agent, Lucia, Lisa, Megan, Anne, Jessica, Miriam, Sophia, and the wonderful staff at Avery, this could not have happened without you.

Thank you, Martha Stewart, for your wisdom; Roseanne Cash, for your generous spirit and elegant foreword; Eva, Arik, Steven, Linda, Gael, and all of the photo models. And a special thanks to Sara, whose lovely presence frequently graces the book. I appreciate you.

I want to acknowledge my staff and colleagues throughout the years for their backing and standing in for me while I wrote this book. And to my patients, from whom I continually learn, bless you.

Thank you, Scott, Allyson, and Ally for keeping me beautiful, Vanessa for capturing us with your photographic eye, and Frank for correcting my Photoshop flops.

And to my furry little Coco Bean, who is no longer here to lick my cheek and toes, you will always be my favorite pup.

Thank you, all. The journey of this book has taken and will continue to take a village. To all, I am eternally grateful.

INDEX

acne therapies, 142, 214–15
AcuFacial® Acupressure Facelift, 37–46. *See also* acupressure regimes
acupressure
 abbreviations guide, 32
 key acupressure points, 229–40
 points to avoid during pregnancy, 37
 pressure and massage technique, 32
 studies on, 8
 Tui Na form of, 31, 35
acupressure regimes
 acne rescue, 214–15
 AcuFacial® Acupressure Facelift, 37–46
 broken capillary rescue, 155
 cold and flu therapy, 125
 headache rescue, 180
 Heart type, 152–54
 Kidney type, 61–63
 Liver type, 178–81
 Lung type, 122–24
 during pregnancy, 37
 principles and benefits, 8, 31–32, 34–36
 Spleen type, 90–94
 sunspot rescue, 193

acupuncture
 acupuncture points, 30
 to improve appearance, 10–11
 for information about, 226
 initial office visit for, 1–4, 227–28
 to select practitioner, 224–27
age spot (liver spot/sunspot) therapies, 193, 194
aging process. *See* Kidneys and Kidney type
allergy patch test, 219
allergy therapy, 88
anger, Liver type and, 172–73

balance and harmony
 in eating, 199–203
 emotions and, 21–22
 overall impact of, 5, 15–16, 21
 through flow of Qi and Blood, 17–18
 Yin and Yang, 16–17
beverages to target in diet
 Heart type, 158
 Kidney type, 69
 Liver type, 186
 Lung type, 130

beverages to target in diet *(cont.)*
    nourishing qualities of, 207
    Spleen type, 99
black foods, 66
Blood, 6, 18, 59
Blood flow. *See* Heart and Heart type
blue light therapy for acne and problem skin, 142
body clock peak times, 23–24
body hair. *See* Lungs and Lung type
body temperature, 200–202
broken capillaries. *See* Heart and Heart type
broken capillary rescue remedy, 155

cellulite therapy, 88
Chinese medicine. *See* Eastern medicine principles
Circle of Life, 6
cleansers, 212–13. *See also* skin care formulas
cold and flu healing therapy, 125
cold conditions, Kidney and, 61
colors
    black foods, 66
    facial skin and foods, 28, 29
    green foods, 182
    red foods, 154
    white foods, 126
    yellow foods, 96
condiments and spices to target in diet
    Heart type, 159
    Kidney type, 70
    Liver type, 186
    Lung type, 130
    nourishing qualities of, 207
    Spleen type, 99–100

dairy foods to target in diet
    Heart type, 158
    Lung type, 129
    nourishing qualities of, 207
dampness, Spleen and, 88–89
diet. *See* foods; recipes
digestion, Spleen and, 87
disharmony, patterns of, 5
dryness, Lungs and, 120

Eastern medicine principles
    approach to cosmetic problems, 5, 10, 14–16
    Blood, 18
    emotions, 21–22
    foods, 27–29
    glossary of terms, 241–48
    Jing, 18
    Meridians, 29–30
    moisture, 18

Organs, 19–21
Organ types, 21
orifices, 27
Qi, 17–18
seasonal phases and elements, 24–25
seasons and times of day, 22–24
Shen, 19
six evils, 26
Yin and Yang, 16–17
eating strategies. *See under* foods
elements, 24–25
emotions
    anger, Liver and, 172–73
    fear, Kidneys and, 59–60
    grief, Lungs and, 116–17
    joy, Heart and, 146
    sensitivity of Organs to, 21–22
    worry, Spleen and, 86
evils
    cold conditions, Kidneys and, 61
    dampness, Spleen and, 88–89
    dryness, Lungs and, 120
    environmental conditions affecting Organs, 26
    heat/fire, Heart and, 151
    wind, Liver and, 176–77
    wind, Lungs and, 120–22
exfoliants, 217. *See also* skin care formulas

facelift regime, 37–46. *See also* acupressure
      regimes
facial care. *See* skin care; skin care formulas
fear, Kidneys and, 59–60
fine lines. *See* Heart and Heart type
fire, Heart and, 151
fish and shellfish to target in diet
    Heart type, 156
    Kidney type, 66–67
    Liver type, 183
    Lung type, 127
    nourishing qualities, 204
    Spleen type, 97
flavor/taste
    balance, 202
    Organ types and, 29
    of specific foods, 204–7
flushed complexion. *See* Heart and Heart type
foods
    balance, 199–203
    Heart type
        eating strategy, 154–56
        foods to target, 154, 156–59
        menu sample, 159–60
        recipes, 160–66

for indigestion, 201
Kidney type
  eating strategy, 63–66
  foods to target, 66–70
  menu sample, 70–72
  recipes, 72–78
Liver type
  eating strategy, 181–83
  foods to target, 182, 183–86
  menu sample, 186–88
  recipes, 188–92
Lung type
  eating strategy, 126–27
  foods to target, 126, 127–30
  menu sample, 131–32
  recipes, 132–38
nourishing qualities of specific foods, 204–7
qualities and impact on Organs, 27–29,
  200–203
Spleen type
  eating strategy, 94–97
  foods to target, 96, 97–100
  menu sample, 100–101
  recipes, 102–8
fowl to target in diet
Heart type, 156
Kidney type, 66–67
Liver type, 183
Lung type, 127
nourishing qualities, 204
Spleen type, 97
fruits to target in diet
Heart type, 157
Kidney type, 68
Liver type, 184
Lung type, 128
nourishing qualities, 205–6
Spleen type, 98

Ginger Oil Hair Tonic, 64
glycols, 218–19
grains to target in diet
Heart type, 157
Kidney type, 68
Liver type, 185
Lung type, 128
nourishing qualities, 206
Spleen type, 98
green foods, 182
grief, Lungs and, 116–17

hair health. See Lungs and Lung type
hair loss. See Kidneys and Kidney type

Hair Tonic, Ginger Oil, 64
harmony and balance
in eating, 199–203
emotions and, 21–22
overall impact of, 5, 15–16, 21
Yin and Yang, 16–17
healing therapies. See rescue therapies
Heart and Heart type
acupressure regime, 152–54
characteristics of, 145–46, 151
eating strategy, 154–56
emotional regulation of, 146
evil, 151
foods to target, 154, 156–59
functions of Heart and symptoms of imbalance,
  20, 146–51
to identify type, 51–52
link to Pericardium and Triple Heater, 150–51
menu sample, 159–60
recipes
  Baked Beets, 161
  Baked Red Snapper with Tomatoes and
    Lemon Broth, 160–61
  Crab and Asparagus Salad with Mustard
    Vinaigrette, 165–66
  Gazpacho Garnished with Fresh Mint, 162
  Red Raspberry Parfait, 163
  Summer Squash Salad, 163
  Tofu and Vegetable Stir-Fry, 164–65
  Tomatoes and Scallions, 162
  Wok-Seared Shrimp with Snow Peas, 164
red foods for, 154
seasons and elements, 24–25
skin care strategy, 166
skin care therapies
  broken capillary remedy, 155
  commercial products, 168–69
  Soothing Face Cream for Dry, Irritated
    Skin, 167–68
  Soothing Face Cream for Red, Blotchy
    Skin, 166–67
  Sun-Free Sunblock, 168
heat, Heart and, 151

indigestion rescue therapy, 201
internal temperature balance, 200–202

Jing, 18
joy, Heart and, 146

Kidneys and Kidney type
acupressure regime, 61–63
black foods for, 66

Kidneys and Kidney type *(cont.)*
  characteristics of, 55–56, 60
  eating strategy, 63–66
  emotional regulation of, 59–60
  evil, 61
  foods to target, 66–70
  functions of Kidneys and symptoms of
    imbalance, 20, 56–61
  hair loss rescue therapy, 64
  to identify type, 49–50
  menu sample, 70–72
  recipes
    Baked Acorn Squash, 74–75
    Dark Fruit Salad, 75–76
    Fresh Fennel Salad, 74
    Lemon Asparagus, 73
    Pork Sausage with Black Beans, 72
    Pork Tenderloin, 73
    Roast Leg of Lamb with Garlic and
     Rosemary, 76–77
    Vegetable Barley Soup, 77–78
  sea salt for, 65
  seasons and elements, 24–25
  skin care strategy, 79–80
  skin care therapies
    commercial products, 81–82
    Eye See You, 81
    Fruits of Heaven, 80–81
    Garden of Eden, 80

LED therapy for acne and problem skin, 142
legumes to target in diet
  Heart type, 157–58
  Kidney type, 68–69
  Liver type, 185
  Lung type, 129
  nourishing qualities, 206
  Spleen type, 98
light therapy for acne and problem skin, 142
lines, facial. *See* Heart and Heart type
Liver and Liver type
  acupressure regime, 178–81
  characteristics of, 171, 172–73, 177
  eating strategy, 181–83
  emotional regulation of, 178
  evil, 176–77
  foods to target, 182, 183–86
  functions of Liver and symptoms of imbalance,
    20, 173–78
  green foods for, 182
  to identify type, 52–53
  menu sample, 186–88
  recipes

    Baked Ratatouille, 190–91
    Dijon White Fish Fillets, 188
    Rock Cornish Game Hen Glazed with
     Peaches and Honey, 190
    Sautéed Spinach with Garlic and Lemon,
     191–92
    Sesame Baked Tofu, 189
    Steamed Mussels in Tomato Broth,
     188–89
    Tropical Fruit Cup, 192
  seasons and elements, 24–25
  skin care strategy, 192–95
  skin care therapies
    Avocado Delight Treatment Mask,
     195–96
    commercial products, 196–97
    sunspot/liver spot therapies, 193, 194
    Sweet Orange Wrinkle Minimizer, 196
    Time-Out Cure, 195
liver spot/sunspot therapies, 193, 194
Lungs and Lung type
  acupressure regime, 122–24
  characteristics of, 114, 115–17, 121
  cold and flu therapy, 125
  eating strategy, 126–27
  emotional regulation of, 116–17
  evils, 120–22
  foods to target, 126, 127–30
  functions of Lungs and symptoms of
    imbalance, 20, 116–22
  to identify type, 51
  menu sample, 131–32
  recipes
    Baked Cauliflower with Béchamel Sauce,
     134–35
    Baked Tilapia, 133
    Baked Tofu and Eggplant, 133–34
    Carrot Soup, 136–37
    Olive Oil and Lemon Dressing, 137
    Poached Pears, 137–38
    Roast Turkey Breast, 135–36
    Steamed Mussels with Shallots and Wine,
     132–33
  seasons and elements, 24–25
  skin care strategy, 138–39
  skin care therapies
    acne and problem skin therapy, 142
    Brown Sugar, Yogurt, and Flaxseed
     Exfoliant, 140
    commercial products, 141–43
    Kefir Cleanser for Oily Skin, 139–40
    Sour Cream Skin Cleanser for Dry Skin, 139
    Strawberries-and-Cream Blemish Mask, 141

sunburn therapy, 138
Vinegar and Lemon Toner, 140
white foods for, 126

Marrow, 59
masks. *See* skin care formulas
massage. *See* acupressure regimes
meats to target in diet
Heart type, 156
Kidney type, 66–67
Liver type, 183
Lung type, 127
nourishing qualities, 204
Spleen type, 97
menu samples. *See under* foods
Meridians, 5–6, 29–30, 32
moisture, 18
moisturizers, 213–15
muscle tone, 9, 86. *See also* Spleen and
Spleen type

nuts and seeds to target in diet
Heart type, 158
Kidney type, 69
Liver type, 185
Lung type, 129
nourishing qualities, 206
Spleen type, 99

oils and fats to target in diet
Heart type, 158
Kidney type, 69
Liver type, 185
Lung type, 130
nourishing qualities, 206–7
Spleen type, 99
oily skin. *See* Lungs and Lung type
Organs. *See also specific Organs*
balance, 5, 15–16
characteristics snapshots
Heart, 146
Kidney, 55
Liver, 171
Lung, 114
Spleen, 84
dependence upon Kidneys, 58–59
emotions corresponding to, 21–22
impact of food on, 27–29
orifices related to, 27
pairs and functions, 6, 19–21
peak seasons and times of day, 22–24
phases and elements, 24–25
six evils, 26

strengths and weaknesses, 21, 47–48
type, to identify, 49–53
orifices, Organs related to, 27

paleness. *See* Heart and Heart type
parabens, 219
patch test for skin allergies, 219
Pericardium, 19, 150
poultry. *See* fowl to target in diet
pregnancy, acupressure during, 37
premature aging. *See* Kidneys and Kidney type
puffiness. *See* Heart and Heart type; Kidneys and
Kidney type

Qi, 5, 17–18
Qi flow. *See* Liver and Liver type

recipes
Heart type
Baked Beets, 161
Baked Red Snapper with Tomatoes and
Lemon Broth, 160–61
Crab and Asparagus Salad with Mustard
Vinaigrette, 165–66
Gazpacho Garnished with Fresh Mint, 162
Red Raspberry Parfait, 163
Summer Squash Salad, 163
Tofu and Vegetable Stir-Fry, 164–65
Tomatoes and Scallions, 162
Wok-Seared Shrimp with Snow Peas, 164
Kidney type
Baked Acorn Squash, 74–75
Dark Fruit Salad, 75–76
Fresh Fennel Salad, 74
Lemon Asparagus, 73
Pork Sausage with Black Beans, 72
Pork Tenderloin, 73
Roast Leg of Lamb with Garlic and
Rosemary, 76–77
Vegetable Barley Soup, 77–78
Liver type
Baked Ratatouille, 190–91
Dijon White Fish Fillets, 188
Rock Cornish Game Hen Glazed with
Peaches and Honey, 190
Sautéed Spinach with Garlic and Lemon,
191–92
Sesame Baked Tofu, 189
Steamed Mussels in Tomato Broth, 188–89
Tropical Fruit Cup, 192
Lung type
Baked Cauliflower with Béchamel Sauce,
134–35

recipes
   Lung type *(cont.)*
      Baked Tilapia, 133
      Baked Tofu and Eggplant, 133–34
      Carrot Soup, 136–37
      Olive Oil and Lemon Dressing, 137
      Poached Pears, 137–38
      Roast Turkey Breast, 135–36
      Steamed Mussels with Shallots and Wine, 132–33
   Spleen type
      Braised Leeks, 104
      Chunky Chicken Soup, 105
      Honey-Nut Dates, 107
      Mashed Medley with Aromatic Spices, 106
      Mediterranean Stewed Fruit, 102
      Mexican Lamb Patties, 105–6
      Perky Peaches with Berries, 107–8
      Rice Cream, 101–2
      Simmering Salmon with Asian Orange Sauce, 103
      Warmed Leftovers and Rice Salad, 103–4
red foods, 154
regimes. *See* acupressure regimes
rescue therapies
   acne, 142, 214–15
   allergies, cellulite, and weight problem, 88
   broken capillaries, 155
   cold and flu, 125
   hair loss, 64
   headaches, 180
   indigestion, 201
   sunburn, 138
   sunspots/liver spots, 193, 194
routines. *See* acupressure regimes

sagging muscles. *See* Spleen and Spleen type
seasons, Organs corresponding to, 22–23
serums. *See* skin care formulas
Shen, 19, 148
six evils
   cold conditions, Kidneys and, 61
   dampness, Spleen and, 88–89
   dryness, Lungs and, 120
   environmental conditions affecting Organs, 26
   heat/fire, Heart and, 151
   wind, Liver and, 176–77
   wind, Lungs and, 120–22
skin care
   acne therapies, 142, 214–15
   broken capillary therapy, 155
   Heart type, 166
   Kidney type, 79–80

Liver type, 192–95
Lung type, 138–39
rituals, 211–18
skin types and conditions, 118–19, 208–11
Spleen type, 108
sunburn therapy, 138
sun exposure, 216
sunspot/liver spot therapies, 193, 194
skin care formulas
   allergy patch test, 219
   commercial brands, 220–22
   commercial product ingredients, 218–20
   Heart type
      commercial products, 168–69
      Soothing Face Cream for Dry, Irritated Skin, 167–68
      Soothing Face Cream for Red, Blotchy Skin, 166–67
      Sun-Free Sunblock, 168
   Kidney type
      commercial products, 81–82
      Eye See You, 81
      Fruits of Heaven, 80–81
      Garden of Eden, 80
   Liver type
      Avocado Delight Treatment Mask, 195–96
      commercial products, 196–97
      Pearl Powder, 194
      Sweet Orange Wrinkle Minimizer, 196
      Time-Out Cure, 195
   Lung type
      Brown Sugar, Yogurt, and Flaxseed Exfoliant, 140
      commercial products, 141–43
      Kefir Cleanser for Oily Skin, 139–40
      Sour Cream Skin Cleanser for Dry Skin, 139
      Strawberries-and-Cream Blemish Mask, 141
      Vinegar and Lemon Toner, 140
   Spleen type
      Bruising Mask, 110–11
      commercial products, 111
      Egg-on-Your-Face Instant Lift, 108–9
      Firming Mask for Sagging Face, 109–10
      Kiwi Quickie Face Mask, 109
      Lemon Lift, 109
sodium lauryl sulfate/sodium laureth sulfate, 219
spices. *See* condiments and spices to target in diet
spider veins. *See* Heart and Heart type
Spleen and Spleen type
   acupressure regime, 90–94
   characteristics of, 84, 90
   eating strategy, 94–97
   emotional regulation of, 89–90

evil, 88–89
foods to target, 96, 97–100
functions of Spleen and symptoms of
    imbalance, 20, 85–90
to identify type, 50–51
menu sample, 100–101
recipes
    Braised Leeks, 104
    Chunky Chicken Soup, 105
    Honey-Nut Dates, 107
    Mashed Medley with Aromatic Spices, 106
    Mediterranean Stewed Fruit, 102
    Mexican Lamb Patties, 105–6
    Perky Peaches with Berries, 107–8
    Rice Cream, 101–2
    Simmering Salmon with Asian Orange
      Sauce, 103
    Warmed Leftovers and Rice Salad, 103–4
seasons and elements, 24–25
skin care strategies, 108
skin care therapies
    Bruising Mask, 110–11
    commercial products, 111
    Egg-on-Your-Face Instant Lift, 108–9
    Firming Mask for Sagging Face, 109–10
    Kiwi Quickie Face Mask, 109
    Lemon Lift, 109
yellow foods for, 96
sun exposure
    damage from, 2, 216
    sunblocks and sunscreens, 216–17
    sunburn therapy, 138
    Sun-Free Sunblock, 168
sunspot/liver spot therapies, 193, 194

taste/flavor
    balance, 202
    Organ types and, 29
    of specific foods, 204–7

temperature
    cold, Kidneys and, 26, 61
    of foods, 202, 204–7
    heat, Heart and, 26, 151
    internal body temperature, 200–202
therapies. *See* rescue therapies
times of day, Organs corresponding to,
    23–24
toners, 213. *See also* skin care formulas
Triple Heater, 19, 150–51

vegetables to target in diet
    Heart type, 156–57
    Kidney type, 67
    Liver type, 184
    Lung type, 127–28
    nourishing qualities, 204–5
    Spleen type, 97–98

washes. *See* skin care formulas
weight problem therapy, 88
white foods, 126
wind
    Liver and, 176–77
    Lungs and, 120–22
worry, Spleen and, 86
wrinkles, 9–10. *See also* Liver
    and Liver type

yellow foods, 96
Yin and Yang
    balance of, 16–17
    cooking methods, 202–3
    Jing, 18
    Organ pairs, 19
    Qi and Blood, 17–18
Yin and Yang foods
    achieving balance with, 27–28, 200
    qualities of specific foods, 67–70, 204–7